Core Fitness

The Body Coach Series

Core Fitness

Ultimate Guide to Achieving Peak Level Fitness
with Australia's Body Coach®

Paul Collins

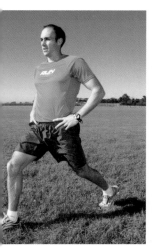
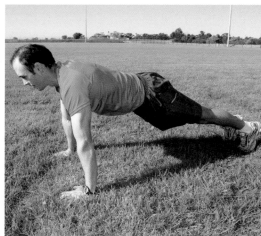
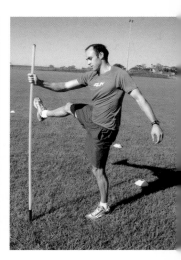

Meyer & Meyer Sport

British Library Cataloguing in Publication Data
A catalogue record for this book is available from the British Library

Paul Collins
Core Fitness
Maidenhead: Meyer & Meyer Sport (UK) Ltd., 2010
ISBN 978-1-84126-292-5

© 2010 Paul Collins (text & photos)
and Meyer & Meyer Sport (UK) Ltd. (Layout)
Aachen, Adelaide, Auckland, Budapest, Cape Town, Graz, Indianapolis,
Maidenhead, Olten (CH), Singapore, Toronto
Member of the World
Sport Publishers' Association (WSPA)
www.w-s-p-a.org

Printed and bound by: B.O.S.S Druck und Medien GmbH, Germany
ISBN 978-1-84126-292-5
E-Mail: info@m-m-sports.com
www.m-m-sports.com

Contents

A special thank you to the following coaches:
Kieran Noonan
Paul Bulatao
Michelle Drielsma
Peter and Michel
Peter Green

Note: Body Coach®; The Body Coach®; Belly Busters®, BodyBell®, Thigh Busters®, 3 Hour Rule®, Fastfeet®, Quickfeet®, Posturefit®, Speedhoop®, Spinal Unloading Block®; Waistline Workout™, Body for Success™, Collins-Technique™, Collins Lateral Fly™, LumbAtube™, Rebound Medicine Ball™, 3B's Principle™, Abs Only™ Class, Core-in-Motion Method™, Abdominal Wheel™ and Australia's Personal Trainer™ are all trademarks of Paul Collins.

About the Author

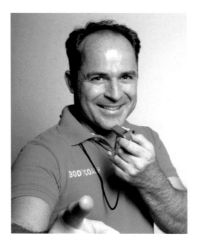

Paul Collins, Australia's Personal Trainer™ is founder of The Body Coach® fitness products, books, DVDs and educational coaching systems – helping people to get fit, lose weight, look good and feel great. Coaching since age 14, Paul has personally trained world-class athletes and teams in a variety of sports from Track and Field, Squash, Rugby, Golf, Soccer and Tennis to members of the Australian World Championship Karate Team, Manly 1st Grade Rugby Union Team and members of the world-renowned Australian Olympic and Paralympic Swimming teams. Paul is an outstanding athlete is his own right, having played grade rugby league in the national competition, an A-grade squash player, National Budokan Karate Champion and NSW State Masters Athletics Track & Field Champion.

A recipient of the prestigious 'Fitness Instructor of the Year Award' in Australia, Paul is regarded by his peers as the 'Trainers' Trainer' having educated thousands of fitness instructors and personal trainers and appearing in TV, radio and print media internationally. Over the past decade, Paul has presented to national sporting bodies including the Australian Track and Field Coaching Association, Australia Swimming Coaches and Teachers Association, Australian Rugby League, Australian Karate Federation and the Australian Fitness Industry as well as travelling to present a highly entertaining series of Corporate Health & Wellbeing Seminars for companies focused on a Body for Success™ in Life and in Business.

Paul holds a Bachelor of Physical Education degree from the Australian College of Physical Education. He is also a Certified Trainer and Assessor, Strength and Conditioning Coach with the Australian Sports Commission and Olympic Weight Lifting Club Power Coach with the Australian Weightlifting Federation. As a Certified Personal Trainer with Fitness Australia, Paul combines over two decades of experience as a talented athlete, coach and mentor for people of all age groups and ability levels in achieving their optimal potential.

In his free time, Paul enjoys competing in track and field, travelling, food and movies. He resides in Sydney, Australia

For more details visit: www.thebodycoach.com

A Word from The Body Coach®

Welcome to Core Fitness

I'm excited about *Core Fitness* for a number of reasons. Firstly, because it has helped me manage and overcome a lower back disability suffered in an accident, and secondly it has provided me with a unique insight into the progressions required to optimize athletic performance – which form part of the 4-Phase Core Fitness Program I aim to share with you!

Core Fitness incorporates a progressive approach to fitness that has you building strength upon strength, skill upon skill and movement upon movement. This approach provides a stable platform that allows you to master one exercise before moving on to the next. It also helps establish important core stability so movement becomes more efficient and the body works as one complete unit.

Society itself is burdened with lower back pain susceptibility through a number of reasons such as:

- Protruding abdomen (overweight)
- Abdominal weakness
- Anterior pelvic tilt
- Lumbar lordosis
- Iliopsoas tension
- Lower back fascial tension
- Gluteal tension and trigger point hot spots or gluteal weakness
- Quadratus lumborum overload
- Imbalances between agonist and antagonist supporting structures
- Poor posture
- Poor muscle control

Abdominal wall musculature without adequate coordination, strength and endurance is more likely to permit surrounding tissues to be taken past their physiological limit, often leading to poor postural habits and lower back tension or pain. With this in mind, *Core Fitness* aims to establish muscular balance, timing and control via more efficient neuromuscular firing of the trunk and deeper stabilizing muscles – forming part of the **The Body Coach® Core Fitness System™**:

- Phase 1: Muscular Pliability and Range of Motion – Warm-up, trigger point releasing and stretching
- Phase 2: Core Fitness Evaluation – 12 Tests
- Phase 3: Core Strength Development – Including 4-Sub Phases
- Phase 4: Core-in-Motion Method™ – Low to High Intensity Movement Drills

In Phase 1, I will guide you through a unique warm-up approach that allows you to reconnect with your body and muscle structure for increasing muscular pliability and range of motion for better core mobility. In Phase 2, there are 12 Tests to help you find your strengths and weaknesses to improve upon. In Phase 3, general core strengthening is introduced along with three additional sub-phases that focus on improving posture and muscle control through a progression of abdominal bracing and breathing drills and the innovative **Cavity-Based Training Approach**™ combining horizontal and vertical strength based exercises to condition the core region. Upon reaching Phase 4, one is introduced to the revolutionary **Core-in-Motion Method**™ (CIMM) with a focus on establishing stamina, strength and endurance of the core region in motion for improving athletic performance. CIMM combines specific training elements that form an ongoing body management cycle that ensures the correct pathway for movement efficiency.

What's more, I have devised a series of Core Fitness programs as the ultimate guide to helping you achieve peak level fitness.

I look forward to working with you!
Paul Collins
The Body Coach®

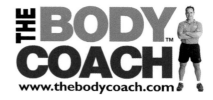
www.thebodycoach.com

Core Fitness Objective:

Optimize athletic performance by building one's core stamina, strength and endurance to maintain a strong core, good body alignment and deep breathing pattern at all times – in multiple planes of motion – whilst performing high intensity efforts over repeated bouts or extended periods of time. Refer to Good Posture diagram and text on page 80.

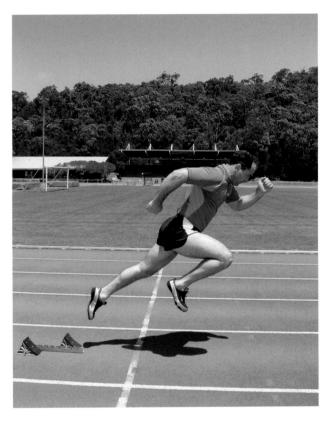

Author Paul Collins in action - maintaining strong core position exploding out of the blocks for the 100m dash. The ability to hold the core for the for the entire distance optimizes his speed potential.

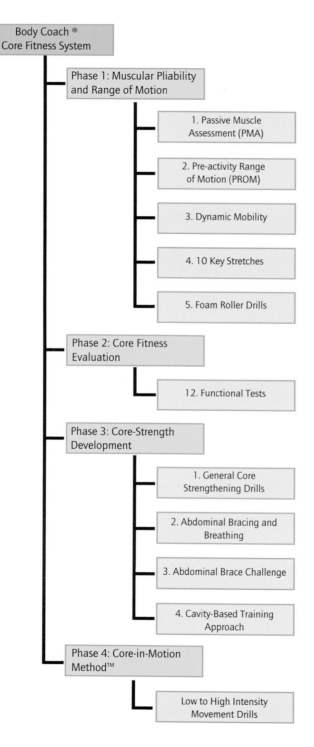

Body Coach ®
Core Fitness System

Phase 1: Muscular Pliability and Range of Motion

1. Passive Muscle Assessment (PMA)

2. Pre-activity Range of Motion (PROM)

3. Dynamic Mobility

4. 10 Key Stretches

5. Foam Roller Drills

Phase 2: Core Fitness Evaluation

12. Functional Tests

Phase 3: Core-Strength Development

1. General Core Strengthening Drills

2. Abdominal Bracing and Breathing

3. Abdominal Brace Challenge

4. Cavity-Based Training Approach

Phase 4: Core-in-Motion Method™

Low to High Intensity Movement Drills

Core Fitness in Motion

Combine the terms 'CORE' (the central or inner most part of body) and 'FITNESS' (good health or physical condition) and you have a functional body in balance for maintaining optimal health all year round.

In light of this, *Core Fitness'* evolves around ones ability to maintain a strong core in movement forming part of The Body Coach® Core-in Motion Method™ (CIMM). Whilst static drills serve a functional purpose, my goal is to build a bridge between static and movement exercises in order to help maximize ones ability to move fast, in different planes of motion, whilst maintaining good posture over extended periods of time. These 4-Phases are outlined in the following flow chart and programs that follow:

Phase 1:
Muscular Pliability and Range of Motion

Objectives

- Establish good body awareness of the musculoskeletal and cavity systems of the body that can affect postural positioning.
- Establish muscle pliability which helps maximize the opportunity for stretching and strengthening with a focus on better body alignment.
- Establish a regular daily warm-up routine to help establish and/or maintain muscular balance for optimal postural alignment and range of motion.

Body Cavities

For the body to work more effectively as one unit, it's important to understand the linkage between the abdomino-pelvic cavity, thoracic cavity, center of gravity, posture and related musculoskeletal framework – larger global muscles and deeper stabilizing muscles. The abdomino-pelvic cavity is based between the diaphragm and pelvic floor region, surrounded by the spine and the abdominal muscle framework which house the internal organs including the stomach, spleen, pancreas, liver, gallbladder, kidneys and small and large intestines. On the other hand, the thoracic cavity houses the heart and lungs. Together, these two major cavities provide the mechanism from which core fitness development is centered based on one's ability to hold and maintain good postural alignment when exercising or playing sport.

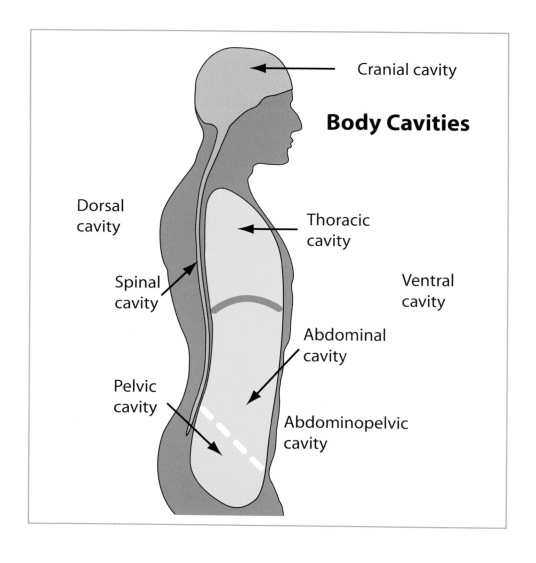

Factors Affecting Good Postural Alignment

The body's internal abdominopelvic and thoracic cavities are surrounded by a musculoskeletal framework that supports one postural alignment. Consequently, weak, imbalanced or tight muscles will affect ones body alignment due to an active insufficiency. Other factors such as lower back injury, excess weight around ones mid-section (obesity), weak abdominal muscles (i.e. childbirth), internal disorders such as Irritable Bowel Syndrome, diabetes or similar can also affect ones posture and muscles firing patterns of the nervous system for maintaining good lumbopelvic positioning.

Good positioning of the spine and pelvic region (lumbopelvic) is vital towards improving athletic performance as it allows the body with the best opportunity to function most efficiently in terms of muscle firing and recruitment in the best postural position. The problem we often face with lumbopelvic weakness is the anterior tilt (forward rotation) of the pelvis causing a postural ripple effect and further misalignment of musculoskeletal structures both up and down the body with rounding of the upper back region, anterior head tilt and inefficient shoulder blade (scapula), lengthened and weak hamstrings as well as tight thigh muscles, gluteal region and ITB, just to name a few. Whilst most peoples body adapt to these positions, they also become more susceptible to injury, especially with high intensity repetitive efforts where one muscle may fatigue as it has to work harder than its opposing muscles. You may also find your body only functioning at 95% of its true potential – so this is where the benefits of Phase 1 comes into play by helping you gauge various muscle groups and release any tension through various trigger release techniques and stretching drills on a daily basis in warming up the body to ensure that any task ahead that ones focus is on good postural alignment and core strength development whilst also re-strengthening opposing muscle groups with muscular balance in mind.

With this in mind, regular weekly sports remedial massage and monthly assessments with your physical therapist are recommended to ensure you reach your goals.

Note: For more information on Postural weakness and abdominal bracing see the diagram on page 82 and Passive Muscle Assesment Diagram on page 16.

Addressing the Issue

Any mechanical disadvantage needs to be assessed and addressed prior to performing or participating in any exercise to help avoid overloading an already over-activated muscle and injury, whilst also allowing you to being able to participate at your optimal level in whatever task or sport you undertake. The objective is towards regaining muscular balance through the regular participation in muscular pliability and range of motion drills as established here in Phase 1 that will allow you re-strengthen the core region in Phases 3 and 4 to help establish good posture once and for all.

Essentially, Phase 1 is designed as a pathway for addressing the issues previously mentioned by providing a warm-up pattern for you to apply. Before we do, let's take a look an one sporting example requiring addressing:

Sport: Rugby Union
Overview: Two x 40-minute halves of high intensity repetitive efforts combined with high impact instances followed by periods of low intensity and stationary recovery.

Issues to Address:
- If the abdominal muscles are weak, the erector spinae muscles can hyperextend the lower back more than usual; the Iliopsoas muscles can also pull on the spine during hip flexor activities which is compounded when combined with hip flexor tension or inflexibility; whilst excessive anterior pelvic tilt can also affect other musculoskeletal supporting structures.
- When abdominal strength or endurance is inadequate to counter the pull of the antagonist erector spinae under load, these lower back muscles are put at a mechanical disadvantage placing additional stress on the very same area.
- In addition, the multi-directional nature of rugby running forwards, backwards, sideways and so forth combined with the impact of the game often lead to deep and upper gluteal tension which can heighten the stress tension on the ITB and TFL which is often a cause of groin strains.

Whilst there are many other additional issues to address in rugby, these alone are enough to keep one busy, especially as they relate to the core region. To help overcome this, postural, movement and trigger point assessments can be performed to address these issues. One key point must be remembered here in that what has taken a specific amount of time to develop also takes a specific amount of time to change. Hence, postural improvements may require ongoing physical therapy, regular weekly massage and daily stretching as well as specific strengthening drills to rebalance the body, especially as we age. This is because strength training performed with the issues stated above would cause a negative effect on the body by strengthening it in a poor position, leading to inefficient movement mechanics. So, whilst you may become strong, it's no good biomechanically if you become stronger with the pelvis tilted forwards, for instance, placing excessive load on the lumbar region. In addition, poor posture can also be caused by poor foot mechanics, requiring the engagement of a podiatrist; whilst poor spinal alignment requires the expertise of a chiropractor or osteopath as well as a nutritionist to keep one's waistline trim and energy levels high.

In summary, Phase 1 aims to address the poor musculoskeletal elements through a progressive sequence of body management drills used prior to and as part of a daily warm-up plan – before a more dynamic warm-up including skills is introduced as part of your normal sport-specific training program. This sequence can also be applied after training or playing to keep muscles pliable, reactive and strong. Thus, when one needs to obtain the correct spinal position or core muscle control in the phases that follow, you will have established the foundation for better movement and muscle motor firing patterns required for improved core fitness and athletic performance.

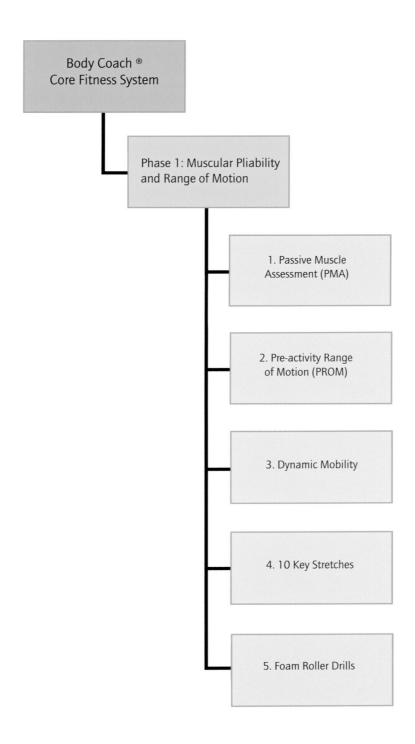

1. Passive Muscle Assessment (PMA)

To help gauge various trigger points around the body, I'd like to introduce you to the term Passive Muscle Assessment (PMA). Tension itself often builds within our muscular framework from the gravitational forces placed on our body, whether through physical activity or a stationary position such as sitting down operating a computer. Many people are unaware of this latent build up of tension occurring over years like a silent time bomb. In some cases symptoms of pain arise out of nowhere causing tension, muscle weakness, a limited range of movement and even reduced athletic performance.

PMA serves as a valuable way for athletes to pinpoint muscular tension throughout the body. The term 'Passive' refers to muscles being tested without function or activity, generally in a lying position using a muscle gauge and release tool known as The Body Coach® Muscle Release Tool (MRT). Emulating a clenched fist or the point of an elbow the MRT allows one to communicate with their body by helping identify and release points of muscular tension.

The key areas MRT aims to address include predominantly the posterior muscles of the body:

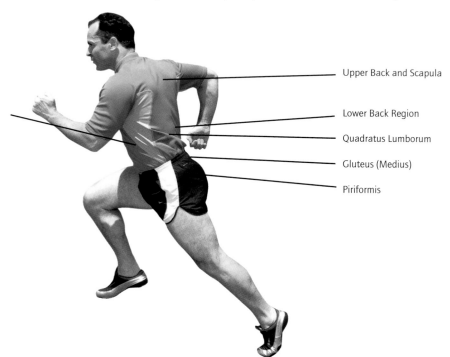

Important note: Weak abdominals can often lead to overloaded and overactive Iliopsoas muscles in sprinting. If this is the case, stretching and massage release techniques need to be applied whilst abdominal bracing and core strengthening are improved to ensure good pelvic alignment and bracing throughout the whole sprint distance at high intensity.

Upper Back and Scapula

Lower Back Region

Quadratus Lumborum

Gluteus (Medius)

Piriformis

On the following pages you will find a series of PMA exercises using The Body Coach® Muscle Release Tool (MRT) to help gauge, identify and release muscular tension. These are especially important for people with lower back (lordotic) arching, anterior pelvic tilt or over-dominant gluteal region:

Passive Muscle Assessment (PMA) Guidelines
- Start with a warm shower.
- Always place MRT on muscle, never on bone.
- Position under muscle and gently add pressure using your own bodyweight.
- Hold position without pain for 5-30 seconds.
- Relocate body position using small increments around specified area.

(i). Gauge and Release Lower Back and Quadratus Lumborum Regions

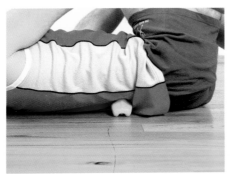 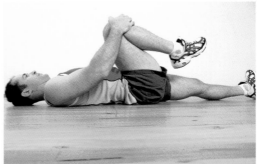

Description: Lie on back with MRT positioned on floor with knob upwards. Lean body onto MRT on erector spinae muscle (never bone). Gently pull knee in towards chest to increase pressure. Release and relocate by moving body up or down small increments. Work up spinal muscles and quadratus lumborum muscles on left and right sides to gauge and release tension.

(ii). Gauge and Release Upper Gluteal Region

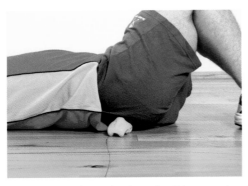 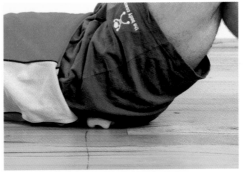

Description: Lie on back and roll legs to the side. Place MRT under upper portion of gluteal region. Roll legs back over to increase pressure and help release any tension. Using small incremental movements, work around whole upper gluteal region on left and right sides to help gauge and release muscular tension.

(iii). Gauge and Release Piriformis

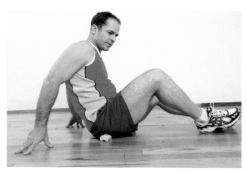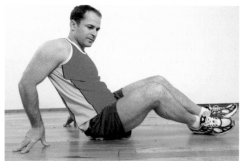

Description: Sit up with hands behind the back and roll legs to the side. Place MRT under mid buttock region and roll legs back over to increase load. Using small incremental movements, work around the whole gluteal region on left and right sides of the body.

(iv). Gauge and Release Shoulder Girdle

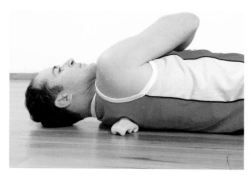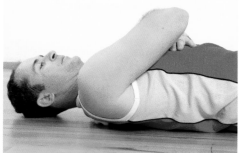

Description: Place MRT on floor with knob upwards. Position body on MRT between spine and shoulder blade on muscle (never bone). Roll body back across to feel pressure. Release and relocate by moving body. Work up and around shoulder blade on both sides to gauge and release tension. Extend arm overhead or raise hips to increase load on muscle group.

For more information on the Body Coach® Muscle Release Tool visit:
www.thebodycoach.com

2. Pre-activity Range of Motion (PROM)

Pre-activity Range of Motion (PROM) is a preliminary series of low intensity exercises performed after a Passive Muscle Assessment (PMA) and prior to any dynamic drills. These exercises provide a long-term benefit for athletes by helping progressively introduce range of motion drills for each joint, bringing body (spatial) awareness, pinpointing any musculoskeletal tension that may require extra attention whilst kick-starting the nervous system into action for the exercises that soon follow.

The objective here is to bring attention to details of oneself and how the body is functioning. The application of PROM drills means that during a dynamic warm-up the athlete will become more conscious of performing each drill with good technique and better body alignment – ultimately leading to establishing proper strength and endurance for improving athletic performance.

At this point it is a good idea to gradually increase the blood flow and body warmth through five minutes of fast paced walking, jogging or similar. Balance, posture, coordination and range of motion PROM drills are then introduced at a low-intensity and slow to moderate pace. Good posture from head to toe is applied along with deep rhythmical breathing. The number of repetitions are kept low, as these are not focused on strength gains but correct muscle control, range of movement and motor control as part of an effective warm-up process. If at any time a muscle feels strain or tension, return to PMA for trigger point releasing or visit your physical therapist for further advice.

The following 8 drills may be utilized as part of a Pre-activity Range of Motion (PROM) Routine.

PROM-1: Hip and Spine Mobility

Description
- Stand tall with feet parallel and hands at chest height.
- Breathing out, gently rotate the body and arms in a flowing motion to the left side, rotating on the balls of the feet. Repeat across to the right side.
- Repeat 8-10 times across to each side.

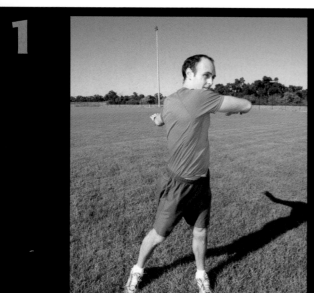
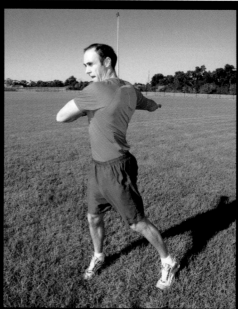

Twist left

Twist right

PROM-2: Body Weight Squats

Description

- Stand tall with feet one and a half shoulder-widths apart and arms extended forward in front of body parallel to ground.
- Lower body slowly by simultaneously bending at the hip, knee and ankle region.
- Keep knee alignment over middle toes and sustain solid foot arch to avoid rolling knees in and lifting heels.
- Repeat 8-12 times.

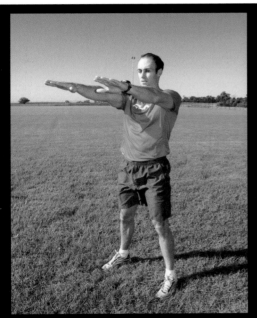
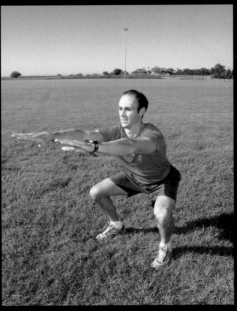

2

Start   Lowered

PROM-3: Stationary Lunge

Description

- Stand tall with one foot forward and leg slightly bent and the other foot back, leg straight and resting up on toes – arms on waist as shown or extended overhead for better body alignment.
- Align pelvis and gently brace abdominal muscles.
- Lower and raise body by simultaneously bending front and rear knee towards ground then rising.
- Repeat both sides 8-10 times (each leg).

Note

- Also perform with arms extended overhead with hands together and body lengthened for increased postural control.

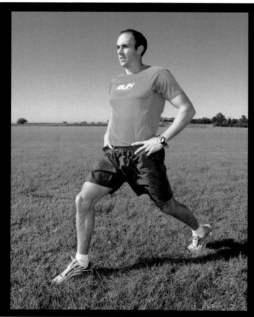
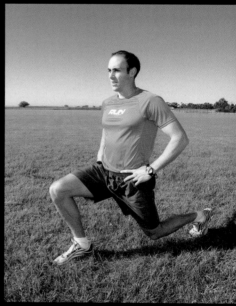

Start   Lowered

PROM-4: Star Jumps

Description

- Stand tall with feet together and arms by your side.
- Gently brace abdominal muscles.
- Simultaneously raise arms up overhead whilst jumping legs out wide, then back together to complete start jump movement.
- Repeat 8-10 times.

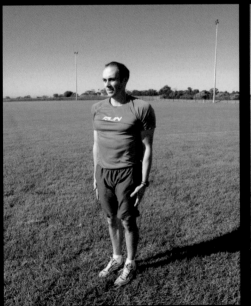
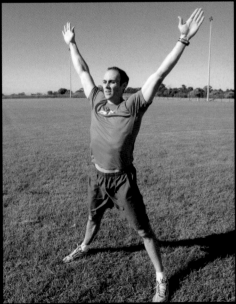

4

Start with arms by side

Midpoint: Arms and legs wide

PROM-5: Lateral Leg Lifts

Description
- Lie on side of body with lower leg bent at hip and knee and head resting against extended lower arm. Upper arm is forward of the body with hand on ground supporting body weight.
- With toes dorsiflexed, raise and lower upper leg keeping the heel as the highest point at all times.
- Repeat 10-15 times each leg.

Note
- For lateral movement in motion see Lateral Side Skips on page 132.

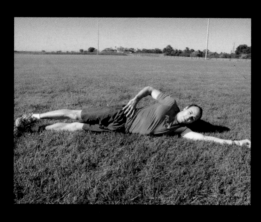

Lie on side

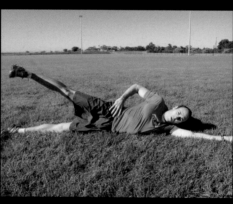

Raise upper leg, keeping heel up high

PROM-6: Push-ups

Description
- Lie on ground in front support position with hands shoulder width apart, body extended resting on toes with feet together.
- Gently brace abdominal muscles holding neutral spine position.
- Keeping arms against body, bend elbows and lower and raise body.
- Repeat 8-10 times without loss of form.

Note
- Perform on knees as lower intensity drill.

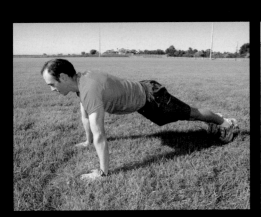
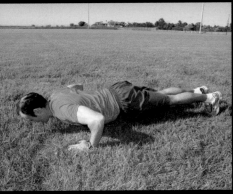

6

Rest on knees and hands   Midpoint: Lower chest to ground

PROM-7: Abdominal Slide

Description

- To activate abdominal muscles that help support the spine, lie on your back with knees bent and rest hands on thighs.
- Contracting abdominal muscles, simultaneously slide hands up thighs until palms reach knees, then lower.
- Repeat 8-12 times.

7

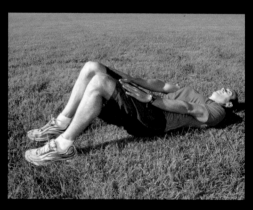

Start

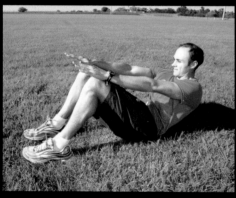

Midpoint: Slide hands to knees

PROM-8: Lower Abdominal Leg Lifts

Description

- Lie on your back with hands under buttock and legs raised vertically though slightly bent.
- Activating lower abdominal muscles, lift hips off ground raising legs up into the air, without swinging legs, then lower.
- Repeat 8-12 times.

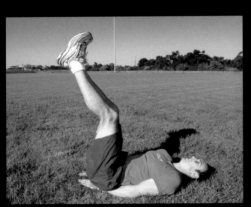

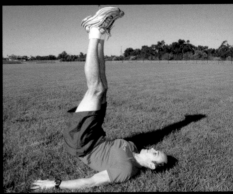

Start   Lifting hips off ground

3. Dynamic Mobility

The next phase of dynamic mobility involves performing a series dynamic stretches briefly for the hip, lower back and leg regions to assist towards ensuring optimal range of motion is achieved. These dynamic mobility drills are performed after a further 5-10 minute moderate intensity warm-up period, such as performing a series 40-60-meter run-throughs at 60-85% of maximum sprint speed with fast walk or jog back recovery to increase heart rate and body temperature.

Post warm-up stretches may include:

DM1: Dynamic Lateral Leg Swing

Leaning against pole, wall or partner, rise up onto ball of foot and swing opposite leg laterally out to side and down in front of opposite leg. Swing across 8 –12 times. Repeat on opposite side.

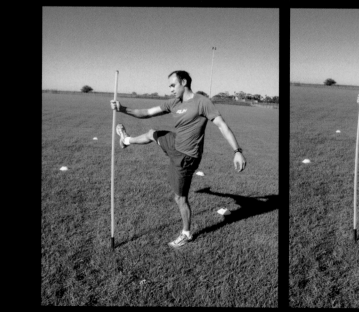
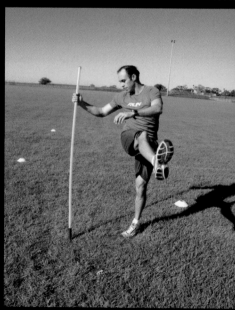

DM2: Dynamic Forward and Back Leg Swing

Leaning against pole, wall or partner for support, rise up onto ball of foot and swing leg forward and back without arching lower back. Keep abdominals braced. Swing forward and back 8 –12 times. Repeat on opposite side.

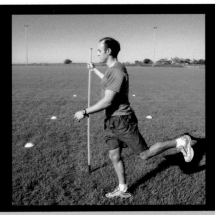
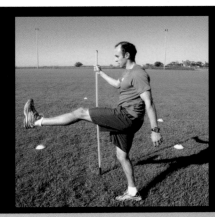

2

DM3: Calves

In a front support position, abdominals braced, rest one foot on top of the other. Resting on toes gently press heel to the floor. Hold 3 seconds then gently bounce on toes for 3 seconds. Repeat on opposite leg.

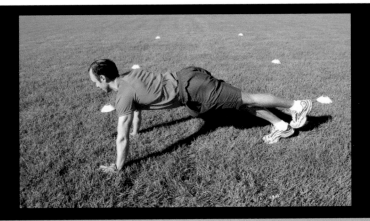

3

DM4: Touch Backs

Lie on stomach on ground with arms wide. Rotate right leg back across body towards ground. Roll back to middle and repeat drill by crossing left leg across body towards ground. Complete this drill in a flowing motion from left to right sides 5-10 times.

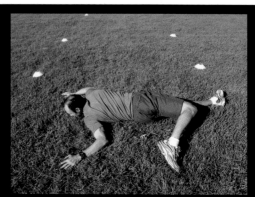
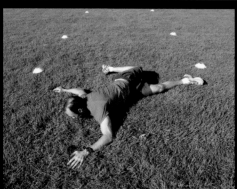

DM5: Crosses

Lie on back with arms outstretched at shoulder height and left leg across body touching ground on right side. Breathing out, draw left leg back across to the midline of the body whilst simultaneously changing legs and taking the right leg across to the left side. Complete this drill in a flowing motion from left to right sides 5-10 times.

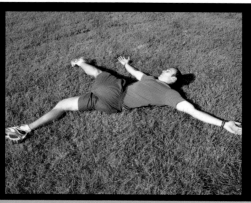
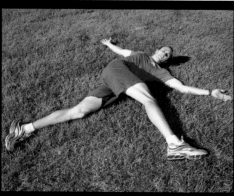

4.   10 Key Stretches for Better Postural Management

After a good warm-up, we now focus on the fourth element – stretching of muscles that surround or attach to the spine and pelvic regions. This ensures the body is warm and free of tension. The following 10 stretches provide a good basis to work from. Hold each stretch or position for up to 15 seconds in pre-activity and up to 30 seconds or more in post-activity without tension or pain. Essentially, pre-activity stretching focuses on bringing attention to correct pelvic alignment and body positioning, whilst post-activity stretching is focused on flexibility. For more information on stretching see The Body Coach *Stretching Basics* book.

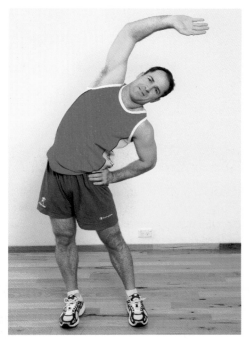
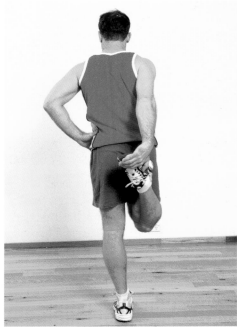

1. Side Bend

Stand with feet shoulder-width apart and hands on hips. Extend one arm overhead and bend to opposite side and hold.
Repeat on opposite side.

2. Thigh

Flex one knee and raise your heel to your buttocks. Slightly flex your supporting leg and grasp your raised foot. Gently pull heel towards buttock. Repeat opposite leg.

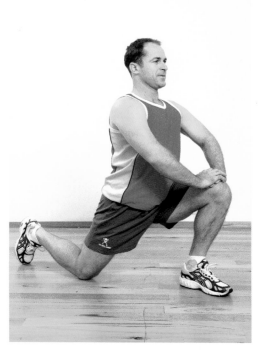 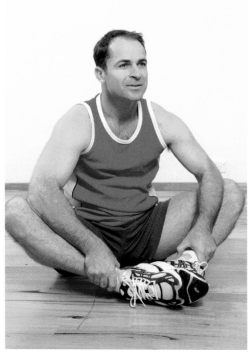

3. Hip Flexors

Extend one leg back, lower body and rest on rear knee and toes. With front leg bent, place hands across thigh and keep tall. Bend forward knee and lower hip towards ground without arching of the lower back. Repeat on opposite side.

4. Groin Stretch

Sit on the floor with the soles of your feet together. Grab both your ankles and rest forearms on inner shin region. Gently push knees towards floor to feel the stretch on inner thigh (groin) area and hold before slowly releasing.

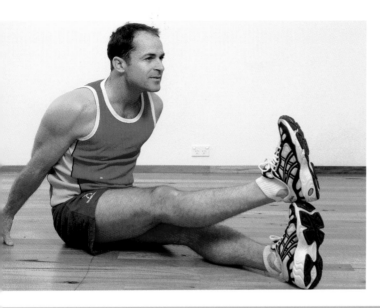

5. Hamstrings

With both legs straight, place one foot on top of the other. Sit tall and place both hands behind the body resting on one's finger tips. Keeping the torso long and tall, gently lean forwards. Go to stretch 6 and 7 before returning to repeat with opposite leg.

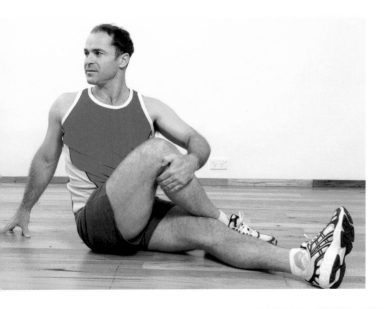

6. Hip, Gluteal and Mid Back

Sit on floor with hands behind back. Cross your right foot over your left leg. Grab your bent leg with left arm and gently twist body to the right side and hold. Repeat on opposite side.

7. Hip, Lower Back and Deep Gluteal

Lie on your back with your left leg crossed over your right knee. Reach right arm through legs and left arm outside, grab front of knee and pull legs towards chest and hold. Repeat with opposite leg raised.

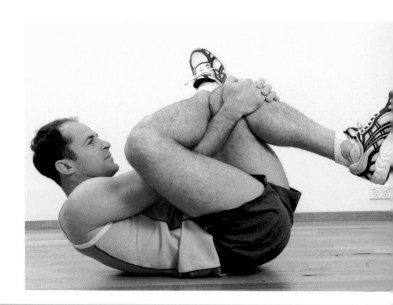

8. Lower Back and Psoas

Lie on your stomach with arms bent by your side and head resting on your fists. Gently brace abdominal muscles and slowly rise onto forearms keeping spine long, then lower.

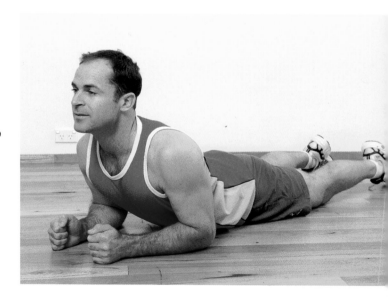

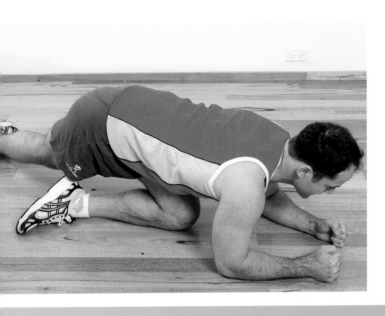

9. Kneeling Sacroiliac Stretch

Resting on shin of forward leg, keep shoulders square and cross one leg over the other, keeping it straight, before gently dropping hip to the side for additional stretch – ensuring shoulders remain square. Repeat opposite side.

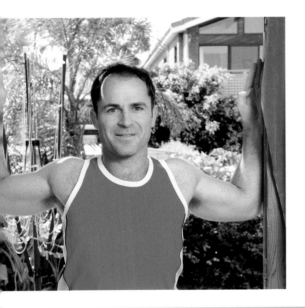

10. Chest Stretch

Find a place between a door frame or edge of two walls. Rest both forearms against wall vertically with one leg forward and the other back. Gently brace abdominal muscles and lean forwards for chest stretch avoiding any lower back arching.

For additional stretching drills please see The Body Coach *Stretching Basics* book.

5. Foam Roller Release Drills

The cylindrical foam roller is a great exercise tool for helping stretch and release muscular tension whilst also helping break down soft tissue adhesions and scar tissue. By using your own body weight on the foam roller you can perform a type of self-massage or what is known as myofascial (muscle and fascia) and trigger point releases as the muscles learn to relax. As you roll over a tender part of the body, allow the muscles to relax before continuing. Continue using the foam roll regularly, before and after training, on a flat surface to keep all areas relaxed. Below are 8 general exercises to get started. Ensure your core is activated at all times.

1

1. Glutes and Hamstrings

Sit on foam roller on the soft, meaty region of your buttock with your hands behind your body. Slowly roll along the foam roller, down your leg toward the back of your knee and back again. Pause on any tight or sore spots. Vary angles of rolling on leg to work the entire muscle.

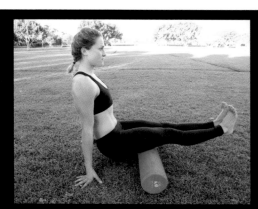

2

2. Thigh

Lie face down on your elbows with the foam roller under the front of your upper leg (thighs). Roll from the bottom of your pelvis to just above your knee and back. You can perform this exercise with one or both legs on the roller, depending upon how much pressure you desire. Vary angles of rolling on leg to work the entire muscle group.

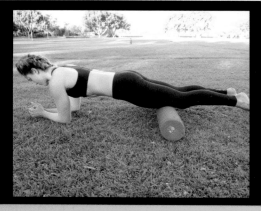

3. IT Band

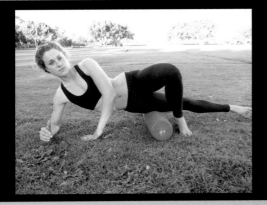

3

Lie on the foam roller on your side, just below the hip. Bend the upper leg for balance and place both hands on ground for support. Roll from the hip down towards your knee, pausing on any tight or sore spots. Repeat on your other leg. For more pressure place your top leg line with the bottom leg and roll. Note: If your IT Band is tight, this may initially feel uncomfortable to perform.

4. Calves

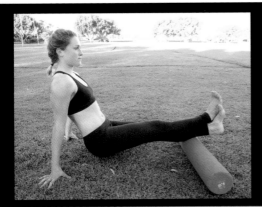

4

Support your weight with your hands behind your body and one calf muscle resting on the foam roller and the other crossed over the top. Do not sit on the floor, instead use your upper body to help roll from your heel to the top of your calf. Alternate legs.

5

5. Upper Back

Lie on the foam roller beneath your shoulder blade so that your spine is perpendicular with the roller. Place your hands behind your head. Bend your knees and lift your hips off the ground. Roll back and forth from the top of the shoulder region down to the bottom of the rib cage to help improve the mobility of the thoracic spine. Use your feet to control your motion and pressure, pausing at any sore spots.

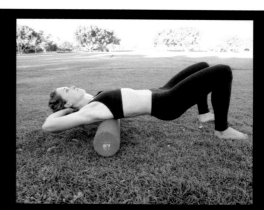

6

6. Latissimus Dorsi, Triceps, Teres Major

To work the latissimus dorsi, teres major and the triceps, lie on your side, with your arm outstretched and the foam roller positioned under your armpit (just at base of the shoulder blade). Slowly roll upward, toward the armpit, pausing at any sore spots. Roll back down and go over again. Repeat on opposite side of the body. Vary angles of rolling to work the entire muscle region.

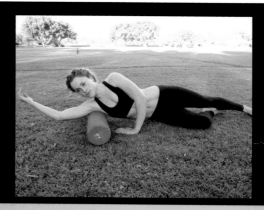

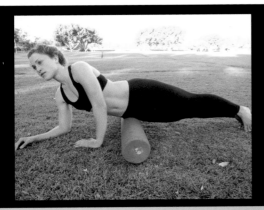

7. TFL Roll

7

The tensor fasciae latae (TFL) is a muscle that runs from the hip to the top of the pelvis. To release this small area, lie on your side so that the foam roller is placed just above the hip joint – just above the bony part of the hip and below the pelvis. Movements are small in nature. Slightly vary your angle lying on top of roller to target this area.

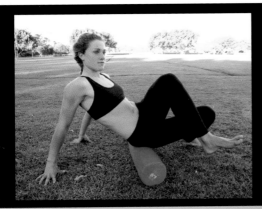

8. Glute Roll

8

Sit on foam roller on one side, resting on glute area with one leg crossed over the other – supported by hands behind the body. From this position, slowly move across roller to release this region. Vary angles of rolling to work the entire muscle region pausing at any sore spots. Repeat on opposite side.

Fore more information on the foam roller visit: www.thebodycoach.com

Phase 2:
Core Fitness Evaluation

Objectives

- Evaluate one's ability to hold a strong core position and ongoing breathing pattern whilst performing a range of exercises that challenge the core through different planes of motion and intensity levels.
- Establish an understanding of strengths and weaknesses throughout the body that need to be improved.
- Provide essential feedback on body positioning, motor skills and breathing.

© fotolia

Core Fitness Evaluation

The core fitness evaluation is designed to help you understand what developmental level you currently hold in terms of core strength and muscular coordination. Assessing, identifying and recording core fitness with various drills provides the appropriate feedback for designing training sessions relative to one's ability level as well as the direction and motivation for improving performance levels.

Essentially every drill is a test within itself, because each exercise can be trained and improved. So, no matter where you stand today, this can certainly be improved in the future. The evaluations I have included are a mixture of drills that require body awareness, stability, core strength, upper and lower body strength and power. In all instances, complete focus and concentration is required by maintaining good form and deep breathing patterns at all times applying the 3B's Principle™ (from page 79).

A muscular-skeletal postural evaluation by a physical therapist is recommended prior to undertaking this core fitness evaluation as muscle weakness or tension or agonist and antagonist imbalances can lead to improper movement mechanics. Your physical therapist will also be able to tell you what tests and exercises are suitable for you.

A proper warm-up period, as provided in Phase 1, is recommended prior to undertaking any core fitness evaluations. The following tests will require a qualified coach or trainer to ensure correct technique is held and unbiased feedback on performance is given. This should be taken as constructive criticism if you are to improve. On the following pages is a list of more than 12 core fitness evaluations to consider. In all instances, abdominal muscle function and strength is crucial towards the ability to stabilize the lower back and prepare for movement, particularly when surfaces are unstable or there are sudden and unexpected changes of direction and force such as those found in many sporting environments.

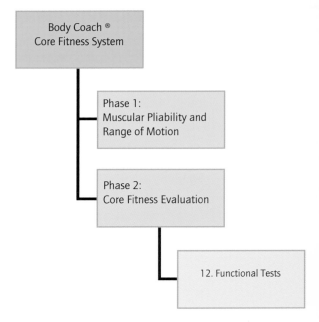

Body Coach ®
Core Fitness System

Phase 1:
Muscular Pliability and
Range of Motion

Phase 2:
Core Fitness Evaluation

12. Functional Tests

Test 1. Body Control: Front Support Raise

Aim: Assess core control in long lever front support position.

Instruction
- Start in a front support position with eye line positioned over fingers and abdominal muscles braced.
- Coach kneels on ground and scoops hands under both ankles.
- Prior to the lift, the athlete contracts abdominal core muscles.
- The coach slowly lifts the legs off the ground until parallel to ground.
- The athlete leans forward keeping shoulders over hands as the coach lifts so as to maintain a tight body position.
- The athlete keeps shoulders forward over hands whilst being raised, ensure bracing and breathing is maintained at all times.
- Coach holds legs for 5-30 seconds, then lowers.
- The athlete needs to maintain a tight body position until the feet touch the ground and the coach releases the legs – no sooner.
- Ensure deep breathing is maintained at all times.

Assessment:
- Upon initiation of the lift, there should be no arching of the lower back by the athlete at all. If so, by any small means, lower the legs and feet to ground and have the athlete reset themselves.
- It is highly important that the coach watch the lower back region at all times when lifting or holding the legs to assess, because this is the key indicator of core weakness.
- If at any time during the lift or hold the lower back arches, the exercise is stopped.
- The athlete should never feel pain in the lumbar region, if so STOP the exercise and lower.
- If the athlete is unable to hold lower back and core stability test by lifting from the feet, shorten the lever and lift under the knees.

Note
- This test can also be performed with the coach holding one leg and lifting to enforce the athlete to contract the whole body.

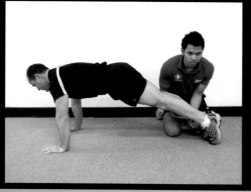

Start Position

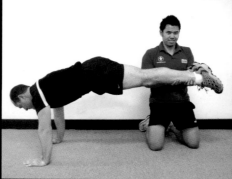

Test Midpoint – maintain core control at all times

Test 2. Body Control: Rear Support Raise

Aim: Assess core control in long lever rear support position.

Instruction
- Lie on your back with legs together, toes pointed and arms extended out to the side.
- Coach kneels on ground and scoops hands under both ankles.
- Prior to the lift, the athlete contracts abdominal core muscles.
- The coach slowly lifts the legs off the ground until at approximately a 30-to-45-degree angle.
- Coach holds legs for 5-30 seconds, then lowers.
- The athlete needs to maintain a tight body position from the shoulders to the feet until the feet touch the ground and the coach releases the legs – no sooner.
- Ensure deep breathing is maintained at all times.

Assessment:
- Upon initiation of the lift, there should be no sagging or bending by the athlete at all. If so, by any small means, lower the legs and feet to ground and have the athlete reset themselves and focus.
- The body should become like a plank of wood from the shoulders (which act as a hinge joint) right through to the feet.
- It is highly important that the coach watch the lower back region at all times when lifting or holding the legs to assess, because this is the key indicator of core weakness.
- If at any time during the lift or hold the lower back or hip region drops or sags, the exercise is stopped.
- The athlete should never feel pain in the lumbar region, if so STOP the exercise and lower.
- Ultimately, the athlete needs to maintain a strong abdominal brace to ensure limited stress on the lower back region as well as deep breathing pattern.
- If the athlete is unable to hold lower back and core stability test by lifting from the feet, shorten the lever and lift under the knees with one hand under the lower back for support to ensure correct body position achieved. This is a great training tip.

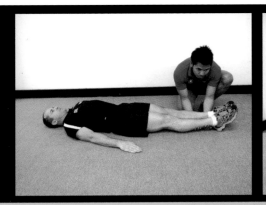

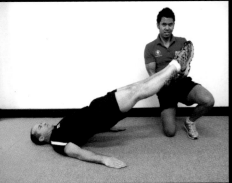

Start Position   **Test Midpoint – maintain core control at all times**

Test 3: Muscular Core Strength: Supine Dish Hold

Aim: Assess co-activation of abdominal core and hip flexors in extended rear support position. As a coach, I have found the Supine Dish Hold as one of the most effective testing and training exercises for improving core-abdominal strength. The reason being relates to the co-activation and firing of the whole rectus abdominus and obliques in line with the hip flexors whilst the athlete has to maintain a strong abdominal brace and deep breathing pattern. In addition, rotational patterns can be introduced for increasing body awareness and the Core-in-Motion Method™ (CIMM).

Instruction
- Lie in an extended position – legs together, toes pointed; arms overhead, hands together.
- Simultaneously brace your core abdominal region and body musculature – raising the arms, shoulders and legs off the ground into a body dish (banana type) position and holding.
- Ensure deep breathing and strong abdominal brace is maintained for a set period of time (i.e. 5-30 seconds or more) without the lower back arching.

Assessment
- If at any time the lower back begins to arch, generally as an occurrence of the arms or legs or abdominals fatiguing, stop the exercise.
- Record the length of time the athlete can hold good form.
- Correct body position is a good indicator of core body strength and muscle control when performing exercises such as push-ups and pull-ups.

Variations of the dish hold include:
- Hand placement – by side of body and raised or folded across chest.
- Leg position – one leg bent and one leg raised (beginner) with arms.

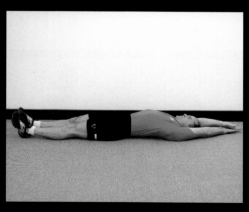

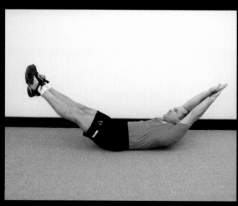

Extended Supine Position   Raised Dish Hold Position

Test 4. Muscular Core Strength: Prone Dish Hold

Aim: Assess co-activation of abdominal core, hip flexors, shoulder and lat regions in extended front support position.

An extension to the challenge of the supine dish hold is the reverse position referred to as the prone dish hold.

Instruction

- Start in a front support position on hands with toes pointed.
- For beginners, rest pointed toes against a wall.
- Keeping the body tight, slide hands forward 15cm or so and hold for five seconds, whilst breathing deeply.
- From here slide arms further forwards onto toenails of feet whilst keeping head down. Limit arm range extended to suit current strength ability through shoulders and abdominal region.
- Maintain dish position and abdominal brace until you lose form (lower back sags or arms fatigue). Stop the exercise by sliding to the ground.
- Assess length of time held in strong dish position.

Note

- The athlete should never feel pain, if so STOP the exercise and lower. Ensure head and neck alignment is maintained at all times with the rest of the body for the development of good posture.

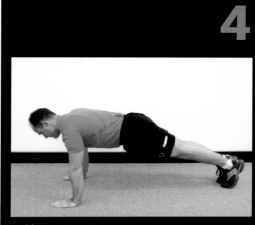

Position 1 – Front Support

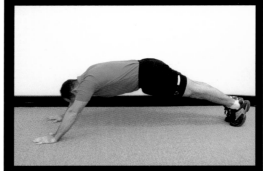

Position 2 – Extend Arms

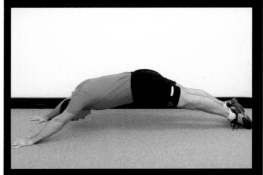

Position 3 – Arms Extend Outwards (advanced level only)

- Limit arm range to suit current strength ability.
- Beginners only perform Positions 1 and 2.
- More advanced athletes can advance to Position 3.

Test 5. Core-by-Association Drill A: Chin-up

Aim: Assess co-activation of abdominal core with the back and arms muscles whilst performing a chin-up.

There is one key element of a chin-up often overlooked – the co-activation of the abdominal muscles to form a dish position whilst raising up and lowering. As the arms pull, one's abdominal muscles are required to co-activate forming a dish position during the pull phase and lowering.

Instruction
- On a high bar with body fully extended, adapt a wide overhand grip (thumbs inward), arms extended.
- Breathe out as you pull up towards the bar.
- For unity to occur from proper core strengthening, as pull ups are performed the abdominal muscles are contracted like that of a supine dish hold on page 44.
- Does this occur – Yes or No.
- Hold position briefly at the top, then lower breathing in.
- Repeat and test ability to activate for a certain amount of reps to show good core strength by association.

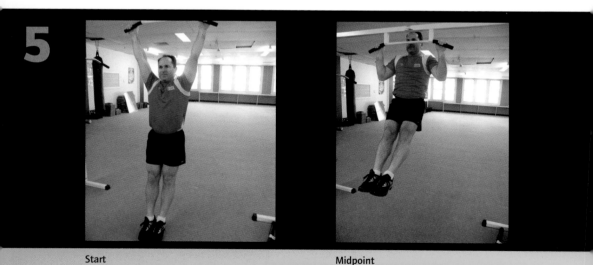

5

Start   Midpoint

Test 6. Core-by-Association Drill B: Push-up (toes pointed)

Aim: Assess co-activation and endurance of abdominal core and pelvic region in a front support position whilst performing a push-up.

Whilst push-ups are generally used to determine an athlete's upper body strength and endurance, it's the appropriate biomechanics of the pelvic region whilst performing a push-up which is of interest here. The purpose behind its inclusion is to measure the athlete's ability to control their upper body weight while stabilizing their shoulder, neck, spine, pelvis and core-abdominal muscles. In other words, the upper body should fatigue before the pelvic region sags or lower back arches (for a set amount of repetitions or set time on task). The core-association is established by the legs being extended and toes pointed resting on the ground on the toenails themselves requiring the abdomen to fire and brace at all times.

Instruction
* Start in a front support position – hands positioned directly under shoulders; body leaning slightly forward with eye line directly over fingernails; abdominal muscles braced; toes pointed resting on toenails.
* Breathing in, bend at the elbows and slowly lower the body towards the ground.
* Keeping the arms close to the body, breathe out as you straighten the arms.

Assessment
* Ensure neutral spine position of head and neck and lumbar region is maintained from strong abdominal brace to avoid lower back sagging.
* The arms should fatigue prior to the lower back or pelvis sagging over set number of repetitions or time to show good core strength by association.

6

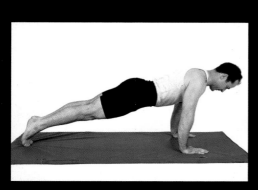
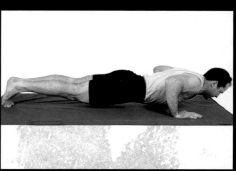

Starting Position   **Midpoint**

Test 7. Squat Patterning

Aim: Assess motor coordination and body alignment (technical) positions in performing a body weight squat.

The squat exercise is the foundation movement for a wide variety of sporting skills from exploding out of the blocks in the 100m dash to jumping, landing and stepping. The squat itself is a highly effective measure of muscular balance, coordination and flexibility due to the requirement of depth, control and body positioning.

Squats are required to be completed in a biomechanically efficient technique, including thighs reaching below parallel to the ground, feet flat with knees aligned over toes whilst maintaining a natural spinal movement pattern. The squat test indicates ability in a combination of muscular control and flexibility. Once a good squat pattern is obtained, a weight training plan can be introduced to strengthen this movement pattern.

A.   Squat Mechanics

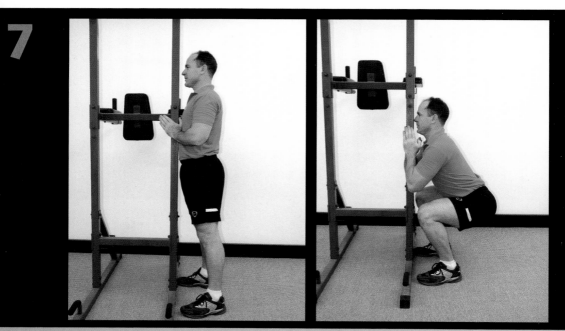

7

Hold pole for support   Slide hands down pole for support

- Stand in front of a pole (or doorframe) with feet aligned at base, shoulder-width apart
- Maintain normal squat position using hands to support movement until body is aligned and balanced.
- The objective is to lower the body by bending the knees, ankle and hips simultaneously whilst keeping the head close to pole – without any faults or restrictions when lowering and raising.
- Ensure feet are flat and knees aligned over toes (without rolling in).
- The hands are used for 3-5 repetitions after which an additional 3-5 reps are performed with the hands held slightly away from pole and only for support if falling backwards.

ASSESSMENT

- With the feet shoulder-width apart and feet slightly splayed at a 15-degree angle, the objective is for the knees to follow the line of the middle toes when lowering or raising without the heels lifting or knees rolling inwards. At the same time, keeping the head close to the pole allows for correct mechanics to occur throughout the body and spine.
- This drill is also a great way to teach the squat exercise as well as a useful warm-up drill prior to exercising – developing muscle synergy, timing and range of motion.
- Ensure breathing in on the way down and out on the way up.
- The restriction of the pole teaches correct movement mechanics which should be imitated when moving away from the pole in the next test that follows.

B.   Supported Single Leg Squat

Aim: Assess motor coordination, body alignment (technical) positions and pelvic position in performing a single leg body weight squat.

Instruction
- Stand tall next to pole and grip with both hands (for initial support) – extending one leg forward.
- Breathe in whilst simultaneously bending the hip, knee and ankles and slowly lowering the body until approximately a 90-degree knee angle.
- Breathing out, raise up to start position.
- The hands are used for 3-5 repetitions after which an additional 3-5 reps are performed with the hands and arms extended forwards.
- Repeat opposite leg.

ASSESSMENT
- Maintain neutral balance through shoulder, knees and feet.
- Assess pelvic positioning in line with leg strength – no sideways tilting.
- Assess lowering point before loss of good mechanics.
- Ensure both legs are balanced. This will further be evaluated in Test 11.

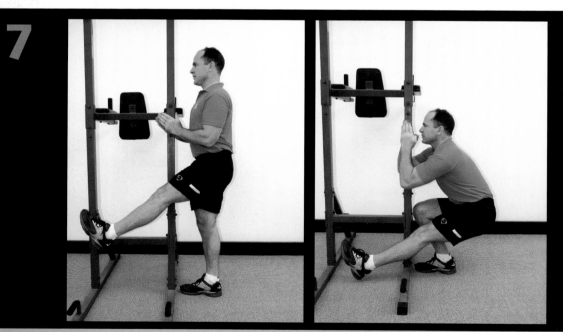

7

Start   Midpoint

Test 8. Squat Power: Standing Long Jump

Aim: Assess motor coordination, core control and power whilst performing a standing long jump for distance.

Squat power is strength multiplied by velocity (speed) driven by the legs and powered through the core and arms. The basis of including this test relies on the fact that some sports are very specific in nature requiring one explosive movement at near maximal output. A good standing long jump score requires good joint stabilization of the whole body in order to generate force, therefore this test is also useful to screen athletes who may lack stability and be posing an injury risk to themselves.

Instruction
- Find a flat grassy area or long jump pit with tape measure and coach to measure landing point.
- Ensure appropriate sporting footwear for grip and stability.
- The athlete places their feet behind the line.
- From a static position, the athlete simultaneously squats, swings their arms backwards, then jumps forwards as far as possible – jumping off and landing on both feet together.

Assessment
- The coach measures from the line to the nearest point of contact. The start of the jump must be from a static position.
- The athlete is allowed three attempts with the best distance recorded.

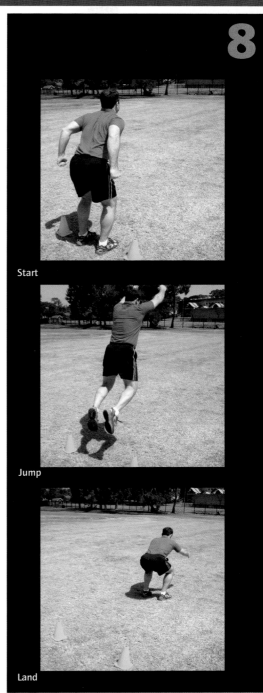

Start

Jump

Land

Test 9. Squat Power: Medicine Ball Squat Release

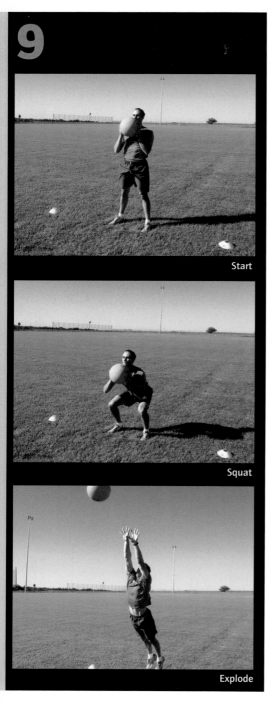

9

Start

Squat

Explode

Aim: Assess motor coordination, core control and power in performing medicine ball squat release to record the distance.

In addition to the standing long jump, the medicine ball release focuses on full body power transferring from the feet through the core to the upper body with a measure of distance of the medicine ball determining core power output.

Equipment required
• Medicine Ball – 3-to-5kg; Open area; Measuring tape and coach.

Instruction
• Stand across line holding medicine on chest in both hands.
• Breathing in, gently squat before exploding the legs and body up off the ground whilst thrusting the medicine ball forwards, away from the chest.
• Ensure you land correctly on both feet with legs shoulder width apart and arms by your side for balance.

Assessment
• Measure distance from starting point to first point of landing.
• The athlete is allowed three attempts with the best distance recorded.

Test 10. Lunge Mechanics A: Multi-Directional Lunges

Aim: Assess motor coordination, body alignment (technical) and pelvic positioning on both sides of the body whilst performing multi-directional lunges.

The lunge is a key movement pattern used in all sports and daily activities in movement and force generation. The Multi-Directional Lunge Test is performed forwards, diagonal, sideways and backwards on each leg. The lunges are assessed for stability at the hip, knee and ankle and for the participant's ability to coordinate and balance the movement. Lunges must be square with no wobbling or loss of form in the lunge and return phases on each leg.

Instruction
- Set up a series of 5 markers in a semi-circular arch one lunge step away from body.
- Stand tall, hands on hips in center.
- Breathe in and lunge forward keeping upper body vertical to forward marker then push back breathing out.
- **Evaluation 1:** Perform one set using the same leg, lunging out and back to each marker – forward; 45-degree angle forward; sideways; back at 45-degree angle; backwards.
- Repeat opposite leg by facing the opposite direction.
- **Evaluation 2:** A call by the coach or trainer can be made to a particular marker to add variety and challenge to the test by being under pressure.

Assessment
- Maintain a strong pelvic position parallel to ground at all times without letting the pelvis drop or lower on one side.
- This exercise can be used as a test of coordination and is good for activities that require multi-directional changes (agility) and dynamic warm-up and stretching.

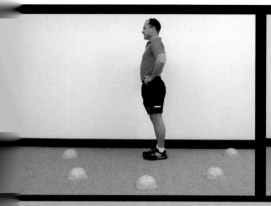

Start and return position

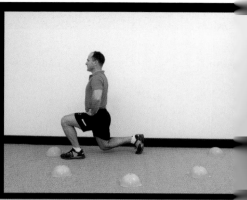

Lunge 1: Forward then back

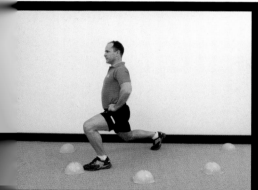

Lunge 2: Lunge 45-degrees

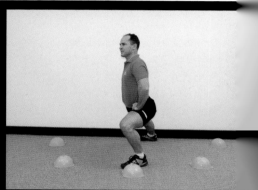

Lunge 3: Lunge sideways

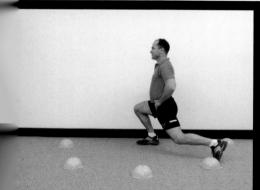

Lunge 4: Backwards 45-degrees

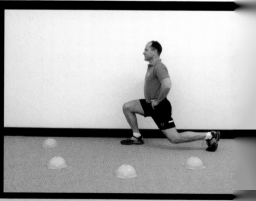

Lunge 5: Lunge backwards

Test 11. Lunge Mechanics B: Flying Start Single-Leg Hop

Aim: Assess motor coordination, pelvic and core control and power in performing a single leg hop on each leg – recording time, number of hops and skill levels.

Equipment required
- 25 meter area or straight line.
- Dry, flat grassy area or sprung wooden floor.
- Markers, stop watch and coach assistant.
- Appropriate sporting footwear for proper grip and stability.

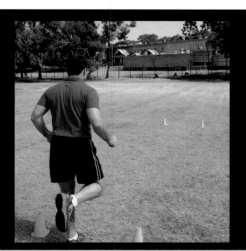 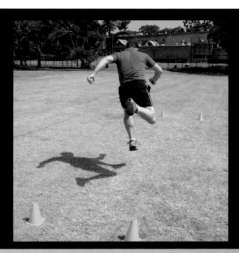

Flying Start   Single Leg Hop 20 meters

Instruction
- The athlete starts 5 meters behind the starting line.
- Using a jogging run up, the athlete starts hopping on the left leg from the first marker.
- The time taken to hop 20 meters between the two markers is recorded.
- Rest 3 minutes and then repeat the test by hopping on the right leg.

Assessment:
1. Time recorded in seconds for:
    (a) Left leg = _____
    (b) Right leg = _____
2. Time difference between left and right leg hop = _____
- Which leg is more dominant – left or right?

3. Total number of hops over the 20 meter distance
   (a) Left leg = _____
   (b) Right leg = _____
4. Hip stability and motor coordination.
   - To monitor the development of an athlete's leg power in each leg, hip stability and muscle coordination.
   - Does the athlete maintain strong pelvic position whilst hopping?
   - Does the athlete have good or poor leg coordination?
   - What areas does the athlete need to improve?

Note:
- This test can be performed over shorter or longer distances.
- Training is adapted to suit the progressive nature of skill, motor coordination, fitness and flexibility.
- The goal of this drill is to maintain excellent body posture, technique and motor coordination, without fatigue, over any set distance, starting from 5 meters up to a maximum of 40 meters.
- If video camera is available, record athlete in action for review and feedback by the athlete.
- It is recommended that the correct hopping technique be learnt in a stationary position using both legs before distance or a number of continuous hops are introduced.

Test 12. Testing Speed

Aim: Assess motor coordination, core control and speed in sprints over a set distance.

Testing of speed is essential in establishing a series of benchmarks to improve upon. These scores can be recorded and referred to throughout the year as a guide to see improvements. The following three tests should be performed on a flat, non-slip surface or athletic track after an appropriate warm-up. The athlete should wear appropriate footwear and sports clothing. A coach is required to start, time and record the athlete's performance.

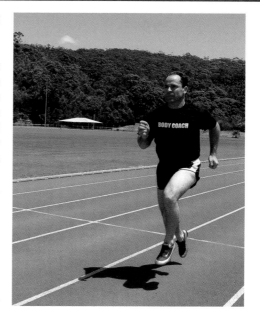

Sprint Tests

Assessment
- Tests can be performed individually or on separate days or with 10 minutes rest between each effort – depending on fitness level.
- Record times in seconds for each distance.
- The main objective apart from time is the ability of the athlete to hold one's core body position over various periods of time at high velocity. This may include filming each sprint for personal awareness of where core weakness occurs and can be improved, especially when one's goal is to run faster.

Instruction
From a standing start record the following:

Test Distance	Time in seconds
100 meter Sprint	
200 meter Sprint	
400 meter Sprint	

Note
- Other additional distances, shorter or longer, may also be applied and tested depending on your training objectives.

Phase 3: Core Strength Development

Objectives:
- Progress the body through a series of four core exercise stages to help establish the necessary core endurance, strength and stamina required for Phase 4: Core-in-Motion Method (CIMM) development.

Core Strength Development

In Core Strength development there is a progression of exercises based upon the type of training outcomes one is aiming to achieve. **General core strengthening** is based around traditional abdominal-based exercises to strengthen and tone the muscle region. To increase body awareness, posture and muscle control, this is achieved through a progression of **abdominal bracing and breathing** drills. A progressive challenge is then placed on the abdominal brace through various strength-orientated exercises involving movement of the arms or legs or both. These abdominal brace challenge exercises include almost all general strength training exercises that require some form of postural control and strong abdominal brace. In other words, focusing on quality of movement at all times without loss of form.

Abdominal wall musculature without adequate coordination, strength and endurance is more likely to permit surrounding tissues to be taken past their physiological limit, often leading to poor postural habits and lower back tension. With this in mind, the previous 3 steps aim to establish muscular balance, timing and control via more efficient neuromuscular firing. Once achieved, this philosophy is applied to the new **Cavity-Based Training** approach linking large compound muscle groups that each require a high level of abdominal and postural focus as the main focal point.

The objective of the cavity-based training approach evolves strengthening of the abdomino-pelvic cavity and major muscle groups for building better body synergy through increased muscle control and breathing whilst using heavier loads. This synergistic approach to exercising involves a push, pull, squat focus. Exercises in this instance include: bench press, military press, deadlifts and squats. Additional exercises can also be used which can be found in my book *Strength Training for Men* as part of The Body Coach book series.

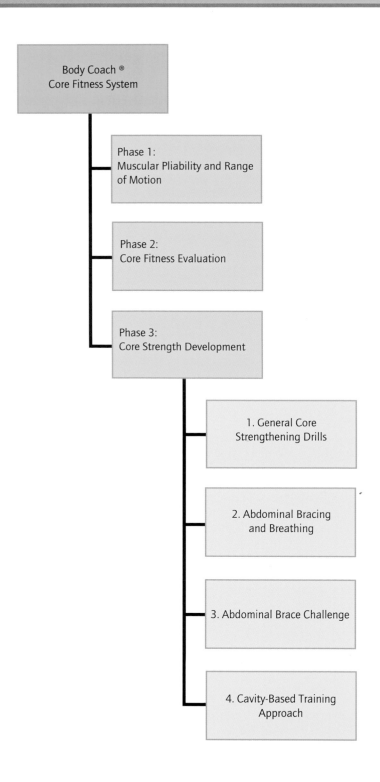

Body Coach ®
Core Fitness System

Phase 1:
Muscular Pliability and Range of Motion

Phase 2:
Core Fitness Evaluation

Phase 3:
Core Strength Development

1. General Core Strengthening Drills

2. Abdominal Bracing and Breathing

3. Abdominal Brace Challenge

4. Cavity-Based Training Approach

1. General Core Strengthening Drills

The abdominal and lower back muscles combine to form the core region of the body. The core region helps stabilize the body for more efficient and effective movement patterns to occur between the upper and lower body and in movement. The following exercises are general in nature and target all areas of the abdominal, lower back and abdominopelvic cavity.

Rectus Abdominus
• Flex the trunk

Obliques
• Rotate, flex, side bend trunk. Support viscera and assist exhalation.

Iliopsoas
• Flexes hip

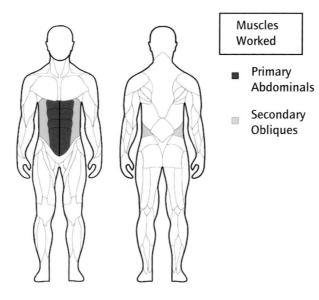

Muscles Worked

■ Primary Abdominals

□ Secondary Obliques

1.   Supine Body Dish

Aim: Strengthening the co-contraction between the core and hip flexor region for better muscle control and strength in a static hold position or number of repetitions.

Instruction
- Lie in an extended position – legs together, toes pointed; arms overhead, hands together. Apply 3B's Principle™.

1. Dish Holds
- Simultaneously raise legs and arms into dish position and hold, ensuring deep breathing and strong abdominal brace is maintained for a set period of time (i.e. 5 or more seconds).

2. Repetition Based
- Lie in an extended position – legs together, toes pointed; arms overhead, hands together.
- Bracing your core abdominal region, contract musculature and simultaneously raise arms and legs into a body dish (banana) position, then lower maintaining long streamlined body position without relaxing.
- Repeat movement for set amount of repetitions with good form.
- Breathe out as you rise up (dish) and breathe in as you lower.

Note
- To reduce the load, bend one leg and raise the other. Alternatively, place both hands on the thighs and slide hands towards knees as shoulders and legs rise off the ground.

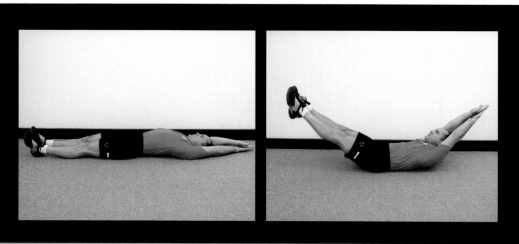

Start   Raised

2.   Medicine Ball Toe Touch

Aim: Strengthening the rectus abdominus muscle for improving muscular endurance of the core region.

Instruction

- Lie on your back with legs raised from hip at 90 degrees and slightly bent. Apply 3B's Principle™.
- Extend arms up above eye line holding Medicine Ball.
- Breathing out, raise shoulders off the ground and reach Medicine Ball up towards feet, then lower.
- Avoid swinging legs or taking hip angle beyond 90 degrees from lower back region.
- Keep head neutral at all times. Avoid leading with chin, use abdominal muscles and maintain good form.

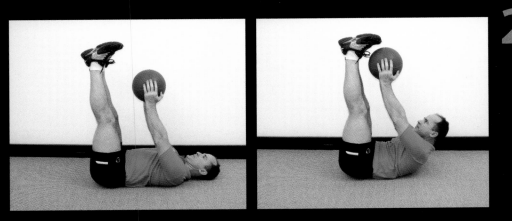

Start   Midpoint

3.   Fitness Ball Abdominal Crunch

Aim: Strengthening the rectus abdominus and obliques for improving muscular endurance of the core region whilst on an unstable surface.

Instruction
- Lie on fitness ball on arch of lower back, legs bent and feet shoulder-width apart. Apply 3B's Principle™.
    - Level 1: Arms across chest
    - Level 2: Hands behind head
    - Level 3: Arms extended overhead
- Breathing out, contract the abdominal muscles and slowly crunch (curl) the stomach muscles up bringing the sternum towards the pelvis. Ensure the ball remains still whilst raising and lowering.
- Breathe in and lower.
- Raise and lower in a controlled manner to ensure tension in the abdominal muscles.
- Maintain the head in its neutral position throughout to avoid neck tension.
- Repeat for desired amount of reps in a slow controlled manner.

3

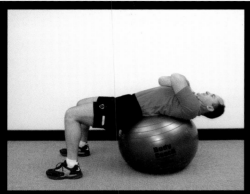

1. Hands across chest

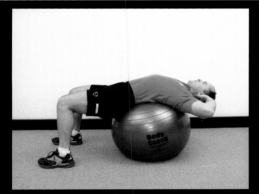

Level 1 - Midpoint – Curl-up

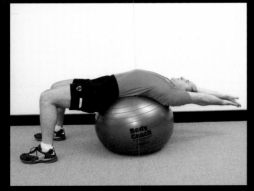

2. Hands behind head

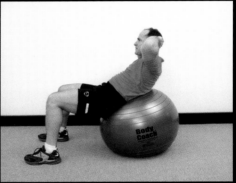

Level 2 - Midpoint – Curl-up

3. Arms extended

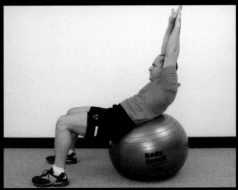

Level 3 - Midpoint – Curl-up

4.   Collins-Lateral Fly™ Series – Long Lever Holds

Aim: Strengthening the co-contraction between the core, obliques and shoulder regions for better muscle control and strength in a static hold position.

Instruction
*   Lie on side with upper body supported by the elbow (90 degrees, directly below shoulder), forearm and clenched fist. Lower body supported by feet – legs together. Apply 3B's Principle™.
*   1. Lift the pelvis off the ground, eliminating the side bending by raising onto the edge of shoes, forming a straight line from the feet to head – Extending arm overhead.
*   2. Extend arm overhead and raise upper leg.
*   Rise up and hold body position for three controlled breaths or 8-10 seconds – left side, then right side.
*   Avoid any twisting or body rotation – keep body tight.

4

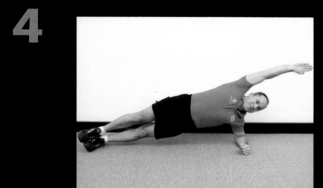

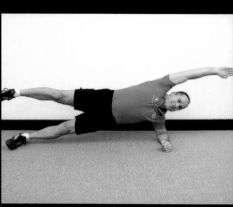

1. Raised Position   2. Raise leg

5. Collins-Lateral Fly™ Series – Coordinated Drills

Aim: Strengthening the co-contraction between the core, obliques and shoulder regions for better muscle control and strength in a static hold position whilst combining a motor coordination challenge from the arms.

Instruction
- Lie on side with upper body supported by the elbow (90 degrees, directly below shoulder), forearm and clenched fist. Lower body supported by feet – positioned together along with legs. Apply 3B's Principle™.
- Extend upper arm to open chest and raise into air.
- Lift the pelvis off the ground, eliminating the side bending by raising onto the edge of shoes, forming a straight line from the feet to head.
- 1. Lower and raise arm as a coordination drill (similar action to chest fly movement, but with just one arm).
- 2. Raise upper leg to increase the challenge whilst lowering and raising arm.
- Rise up and hold body position for three controlled breaths or 8-10 seconds whilst raising and lower arm. Repeat left side, then right side.
- Avoid any twisting or body rotation – keep body tight.

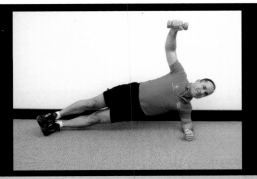

5

1. Start   Lower and raise arm - weighted

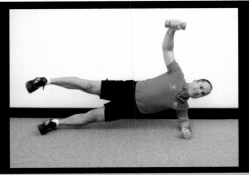

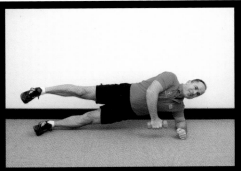

2. Raise leg   Lower and raise arm (weighted) with leg raised

6. Lateral Side Raises

Aim: Strengthening the co-contraction between the upper and lower body through the core region in a side lying dynamic drill movement pattern.

Instruction
- Lie on your side, legs extended, toes pointed and feet together.
- The arm closest to the ground extends above head with palm facing towards ceiling – head relaxed resting on inner part of arm.
- The upper arm is bent, supporting your body weight in front of the body. Apply 3B's Principle™.
- Breathing in through the nose, then out through the mouth with pursed lips, draw your navel inwards and hold – maintaining a neutral spine.
- Maintaining a long body position, forcefully breathe out through pursed lips and simultaneously raise legs and arm into the air, then lower.
- Repeat in rapid motion for desired amount of reps in a controlled manner.
- Repeat on opposite side.

Note
- Maintain tight and long body position by leaning body slightly forward and putting weight onto hand supporting the body. Avoid leaning or falling backwards.

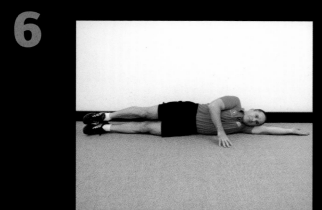

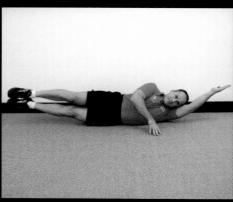

Starting Position   **Midpoint – Legs and arms raised**

7.   Medicine Ball Elbow to Knee

Aim: Strengthening the oblique muscles using an externally weighted medicine ball in a supine lying position.

Instruction

- Lie on your back with one leg bent and the other foot resting on the opposite knee.
- Apply 3B's Principle™.
- Rest Medicine Ball on opposite shoulder to raised knee.
- Breathing out, raise opposite elbow towards opposite knee.
- Breathe in and lower.
- Repeat in rapid motion for desired amount of reps in a controlled manner.
- Repeat on opposite side.

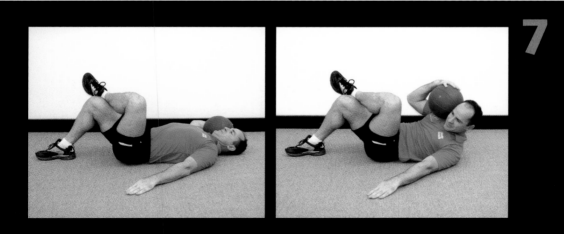

Start	Elbow to knee with medicine ball

8. Lower Leg Lifts

Aim: Strengthening of the rectus abdominus and obliques through lower abdominal leg lifts lying in a supine position on one's back.

Instruction
- Lie on your back with legs raised in the air and slightly bent and hands placed under your buttocks – palms down.
- Apply 3B's Principle™.
- Maintaining a strong abdominal brace, breathe out as you activate the lower abdominal region and raise the hip, legs and buttocks off the ground without swinging legs or changing their length.
- Breathe in as you lower buttocks to ground in a controlled manner.

Note
- Over time, with good abdominal contraction you will learn to relax the upper body and focus on solely activating the abdominal region.
- Repeat in rapid motion for desired amount of reps in a controlled manner.

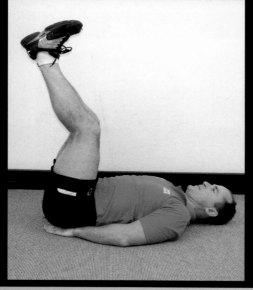

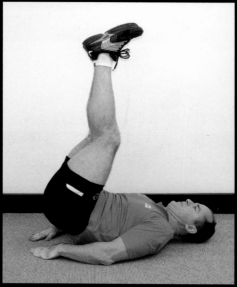

Start   Raised

9.   Knee Raises

Aim: Strengthening the co-contraction between the rectus abdominus, obliques and hip flexors for better lower abdominal endurance and core control.

Instruction
- Position forearms on pads with shoulders kept high in captain's chair (or similar machine) with legs extended down and abdominal muscles braced.
- Apply 3B's Principle™.
- Maintain slight body dish position until exercise set is complete.
- Breathing out, raise knees to chest. Once thigh is parallel to ground, drive knees towards chest to obtain maximum abdominal contraction.
- Breathe in and slowly lower legs to starting position.

Note
- Avoid legs relaxing or swinging backwards when lowering.

Variations
1. Raise and twist knees diagonally to activate the obliques.
2. Single leg straight leg raises until parallel to ground.
3. Double leg straight leg raises until parallel to ground.

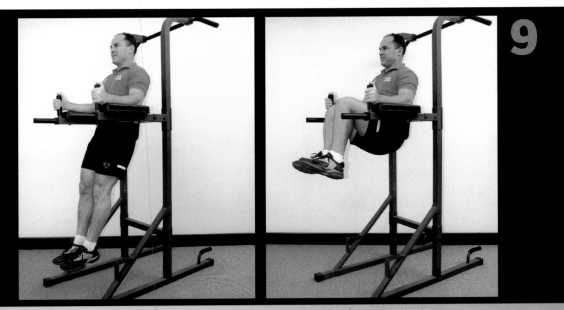

Start   Raised

10. Hanging Raises

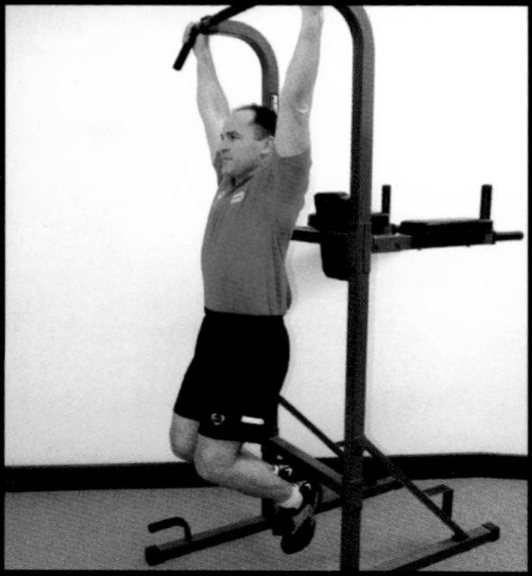

Start

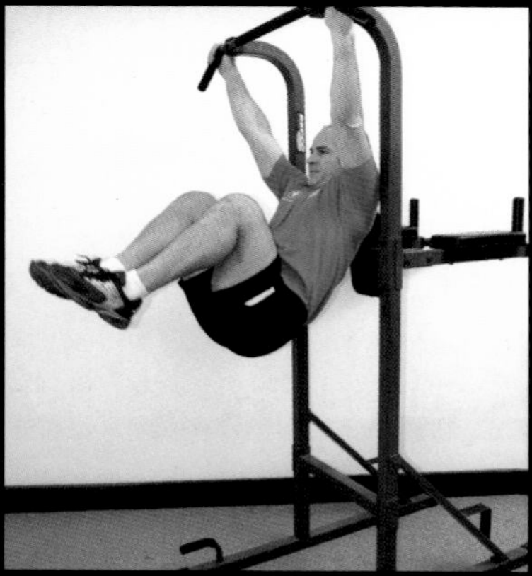

10a. Knees raised

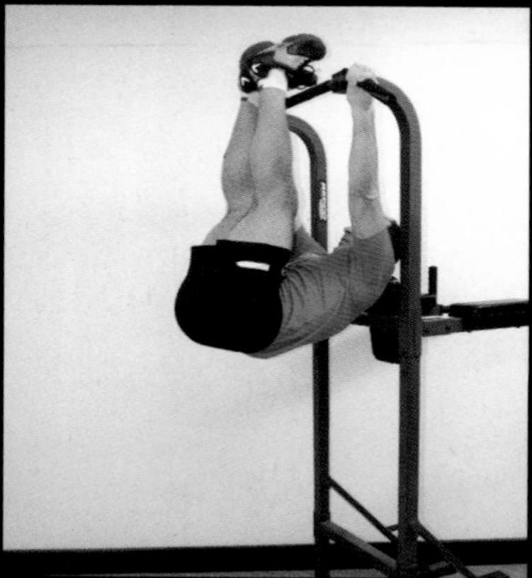

10b. Feet raised – legs straight

Aim: Strengthening the co-contraction between the rectus abdominus, obliques, and hip flexors whilst in a hanging wide grip position for better lower endurance and abdominal control.

Instruction
- Grip an overhead bar with arms and legs extended and brace abdominal muscles.
- Breathing out, (a) raise knees to chest; OR (b) raise feet to bar; then lower legs slowly. Aim to maintain a tight body position at all times and avoid abdominal swinging (weakness).
- Breathe in and lower legs in a controlled movement.

Note
- A coach may be necessary to support the lower back region of the athlete to reduce any swinging.

11.   Pistons

Aim: Strengthening the whole core region, including hip flexors, in a motor-coordinated environment involving the arms and legs.

Instruction
- Advanced exercise for experienced athletes.
- Lie flat on your back with one leg straight and the other bent – feet parallel and abdominal muscles braced.
- Place hands behind the head and twist opposite elbow towards opposite knee – keeping the torso braced.
- Apply 3B's Principle™.
- Simultaneously straighten one leg whilst you extend the other, slightly turning the opposite elbow towards the opposite knee.
- Perform movement in a slow controlled motion whilst maintaining strong abdominal brace.
- Breathe out as you extend the leg.
- Maintain a deep breathing pattern and a tight body position with minimal sideways movement. In which case, the torso remains stationary and small action of the arms increases the exercise intensity.

Exercise Tips:
- Start with slow, controlled motion and deep breathing pattern.
- This exercise should look smooth with the athlete always in control.
- This exercise is for advanced exercisers only who can maintain pelvic and spinal alignment.

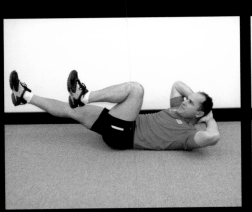 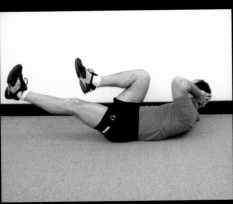

11

Opposite elbow to knee   Repeat opposite side

12.   Hip Bridge

Aim: Support the abdominal muscles through strengthening and activation of lower back and gluteal muscles in a supine raised position.

Instruction

- Lie flat on back with legs bent and arms by your side.
- Apply 3B's Principle™.
- Breathe in deeply.
- Breathe out and slowly peel the lower back off the ground and raise hips into the air.
- Breathe in at the top of the movement and re-activate abdominal muscles. Complete one full breath in and out – then in again before lowering body.
- Breathe out and lower the body in reverse motion lowering hips to ground.

Note

- Balance on heels and raise to introduce hamstrings muscle involvement.
- Maintain square hips at all times.
- To increase the intensity of the Hip Raise, extend one leg upwards and hold. A similar approach is resting on one heel to activate hamstrings muscles.

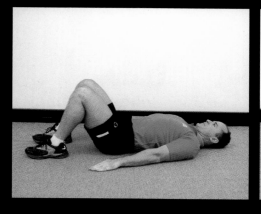

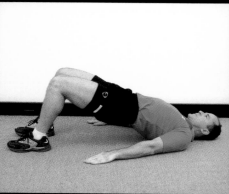

Start

Midpoint – Raise hips

13.   Controlled Back Raise

Aim: Support the abdominal muscles through strengthening and activation of lower back and gluteal muscles in a prone raised position.

Instruction
- To strengthen the lower back region, lie on stomach with hands clasped behind back.
- Apply 3B's Principle™.
- Breathing out, contract stomach and raise upper body (chest) off floor.
- Focus on elongating the spine and rising away and up a short distance whilst maintaining braced abdominal muscles.
- Breathing in, slowly lower the chest back to the floor.
- Up and down for a count of 2.

Note
- No tension or pain should be felt in the lower back at any time during exercise. Stretch lower back in between sets by lying on your back and bringing your knees to your chest.

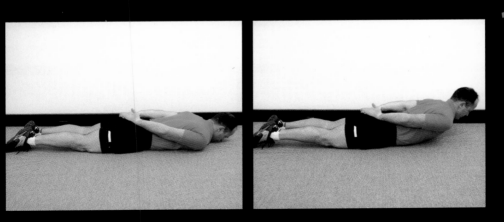

Start   Raised

14. Fitness Ball Isometric Rear Supports

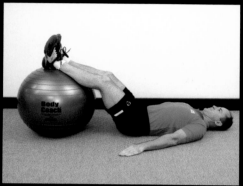

Level 1 (Low) – Arms flat

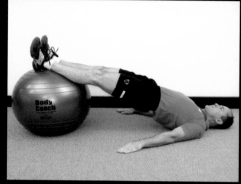

LEVEL 1 – Body raised

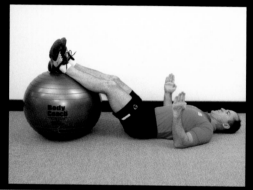

Level 2 (Medium) – Elbows bent

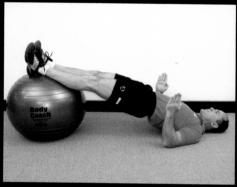

Level 2 – Body raised

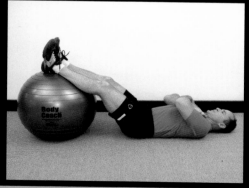

Level 3 (High) – Arms across chest

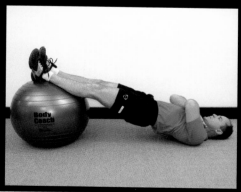

Level 3 – Body raised

Aim: Support the abdominal muscles through strengthening and activation of lower back and gluteal muscles in a supine raised position on an unstable surface.

Level 1 – Low Intensity
- Lie on back, flex at hip and rest feet on ball. Apply 3B's Principle™.
- Extend arms on floor at 45-degree angle to body.
- Breathing out, slowly raise buttocks, hips and back off ground.
- Hold extended position breathing deeply for 1-5 breaths, then lower.

Level 2 – Medium Intensity
- Lie on back, flex at hips and rest feet on ball. Apply 3B's Principle™.
- Bend elbows and rest across triceps with fingers pointed towards sky.
- Breathing out, slowly raise buttocks, hips and back off ground.
- Hold extended position breathing deeply for 1-5 breaths, then lower.

Level 3 – High Intensity
- Lie on back, flex at hips and rest feet on ball. Apply 3B's Principle™.
- Cross arms across chest.
- Breathing out, slowly raise buttocks, hips and back off ground.
- Hold extended position breathing deeply for 1-5 breaths, then lower.

Note
- Have a coach assist all holding patterns with one hand supporting the lower back and the other behind the knee or the ball.
- Ensure a strong core and deep breathing pattern at all times.
- Expect slight muscle shaking whilst the body aims to gain control of the movement pattern, especially Levels 2 and 3 where there is minimal arm support.

Core Strength Sample Workout

Core strength exercises can be performed on a daily basis. Exercises and specific regions can also be rotated on a daily basis, for instance Rectus Abdominus Monday, Obliques Tuesday and so forth. The tempo itself will often guide the number of repetitions performed (eg. 1 second up, 3 seconds lowering per repetition is a lot more demanding than 1 second up, 1 second lowering). Some exercises are more dynamic in nature than others, such as the lateral side raises, although in most instances performing an exercise slower and more controlled will bring greater results. So, once you hit the Core-in-Motion Method™ (CIMM) you will have the essential foundation conditioning of the core region in bracing ability and strength to optimize your core fitness potential. The following sample workout, and others, can be used in combination with the CIMM method during a training week for great results.

Sample Workout:

EXERCISE	REPS	SETS	RECOVERY
1. Body Dish	5-20 second holds	3-5	15-seconds
2. Lateral Side Raises	20	3 sets each side	Nil. Move from one side onto the other
3. Lower Leg Lifts	15-30	3-5	60 seconds
4. Hanging Knee Raises	10-20	3-5	60 seconds
5. Hip Bridge	8-12	3	60 seconds

2. Abdominal Bracing and Breathing

3B's Principle™: Pre-exercise set-up

Every exercise has a number of key elements to consider when setting up and performing the specific movement. None more so than the ability to maintain good posture at all times throughout the exercise whether a low, medium or high intensity load. Applying correct technique from the onset will help establish body awareness and muscle control required for good form which is ultimately maintained throughout the whole exercise task at hand until the series of repetitions (or time) are completed.

Combining deep breathing with abdominal bracing is important because it teaches you to contract your abdominal (stomach) muscles, which play an important role in developing good posture, awareness of your body position in space and time (movement) and protecting your lower back region from being overloaded. Abdominal Bracing holds an important role in most exercises and can be performed sitting, lying, kneeling, standing, walking or in sports specific movement drills.

The 3 key elements required in order to maintain good body position whilst exercising form part of a simple exercise set-up phrase I've termed the **3B's Principle™**:

(1) Brace
(2) Breath
(3) Body Position.

1. Brace

Activation of deepest muscle of the abdominal wall, the transversus abdominis muscle (TVA) in line with the obliques is crucial to the stability and function of the deep abdominal wall and lumbar region. The function of this muscle with other surrounding abdominal oblique and deep spinal stabilization muscles is of high importance during times of physical stress or in sport where impact is involved due to the high level of stabilization required. Activating your abdominal muscles through abdominal bracing prior to and throughout exercising is important because it contributes to spinal stabilization through a mechanism referred to as intra-abdominal pressure within the abdominopelvic cavity, which helps activate the larger global muscles in line with the deeper stabilizing muscles re-align the spine and unload stress placed on the lumbar region whilst increasing awareness of one's body position in movement.

Research suggests that the muscles are best exercised at low intensity, and suggest that levels of 40% of maximal voluntary contraction (MVC) are most favorable. The reason for this is that the stabilizing muscles are postural muscles that work continuously at low levels of maximal muscle contraction. With this type of approach you become more aware of the deeper inner framework of your body over time leading to better core-activation and maintenance of good pelvic alignment.

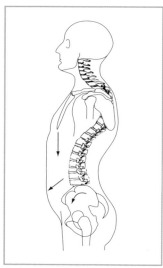

Poor Posture

- Protruding abdomen
- Forward head tilt
- Rounded shoulders and scapula displacement
- Thoracic kyphosis
- Lumbar curvature often causing a lumbar fascia to contract and tighten
- Forward pelvic tilt often results in weakened hamstrings and tight thigh or ilipsoas muscles

Poor posture is contributed to a number of poor lifestyle habits such as obesity, instability through muscular overuse or muscular imbalance and lower back injury. The action of gently pulling-in the abdomen and bracing prior to and throughout each exercise is important because it generates intra-abdominal pressure within the abdominopelvic cavity (pushing up against the diaphragm and down towards the pelvic floor), whilst contributing to a deep stabilizing function through enhanced motor control.

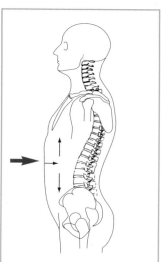

Good Posture
'Abdominal Brace Applied'

Notice how drawing the abdomen in helps re-align the body. One of the main goals of Athletic Abs is to be able to maintain this position at all times whilst exercising:

- Abdominals braced - increases intra-abdominal pressure
- Improved head and neck alignment
- Improved shoulder and scapula positioning
- Improved alignment of the spine
- Improved pelvic alignment contributing to better lower body mechanics

Then through regular training develop a strong core that holds good body alignment and posture at all times

Through the implementation of Phase 1 pre-activity steps and physical therapy treatments and massage on an ongoing basis, this helps reduce the risk of injury susceptibility through increased self awareness, body management and muscular control. It also allows time for the athlete to re-balance and re-strengthen the body's muscular framework for better muscular (phasic) tone and postural control whilst the body is in good alignment. Hence, the importance of a healthy diet and keeping a trim waistline, regular stretching and massage on a daily and weekly basis and dedication to core fitness development as outlined in this book.

If you find when drawing in the abdomen a resistance from the pelvic region to realign (reducing lumbar curvature), you may find that the Psoas major muscles has become dominant due to weak abdominal muscles also causing lower back and ITB fascial tension, overactivation of quadratus lumborum and upper gluteal region as well as hamstrings weakness or thigh tension. As a result, more time may have to be spent stretching with a focus on the releasing the psoas as shown below and practicing bracing drills in examples 1–4 that soon follow.

Psoas Stretch

Note: Only perform this stretch after applying Phase 1 warm-up drills.

Starting Position
- Spread legs wide and lean forward and place both hands on the ground.

Action – Variation 1
- Gently brace the abdominal muscles.
- Turn feet out and rest on instep of both feet on ground.
- Maintain weight on hands and keep arms extended.
- Slowly lower hips to ground keeping head raised and spine long.
- No pain or tension should be present.
- Maintain deep breathing pattern.
- Hold stretch for up to 15 seconds without any lower back tension.

Action – Variation 2
- Turn to one side and raise onto heel of front foot and toes of back foot and lower hip to ground.
- Maintain weight on hands and keep arms extended.
- Hold stretch for up to 15 seconds.
- Maintain deep breathing pattern.
- Repeat stretch on opposite side.

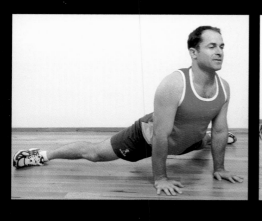
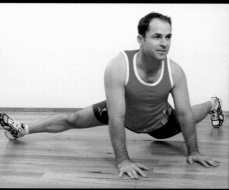

Variation 1   Variation 2

Abdominal bracing drills should first be practiced kneeling, sitting, lying and standing to develop the appropriate body awareness from which a foundation is established and built upon. This is achieved through simple bracing and deep breathing techniques. The resulting outcomes often expressed by athletes include better posture and motor control of the deep stabilizing muscles enabling them to establish a unique inner awareness of their body in space and time and increased movement efficiency and athletic performance.

Example 1: 4-Point Abdominal Bracing Drill

Instruction
- In the four-point kneeling position (on your hands and knees), take a deep breath inwards through your nose, then as you breathe out through your mouth, draw your navel (belly button) inwards towards your spine and hold without changing your neutral spine position.
- Using big, deep breaths, continue breathing in your nose and out your mouth whilst holding this braced position, for 5-10 breaths.
- Relax and repeat for 3-5 sets.

Note
- Example 1 is a great starting point, as drawing in the abdominal wall without movement of the spine or pelvis should be achieved with minimal activation of the larger trunk muscles, whilst deep breathing is maintained. Once endurance in this position is achieved, you can increase the lever length from the knees up onto the toes into a front support position and others as part of examples 2 and 3.
- Start with 5 deep breaths and over time progress to 10 breaths.
- Initially, breathing may feel short and the stomach hard to hold in at all times whilst breathing, but with ongoing practice you will improve your ability to brace and breathe more efficiently, without contracting other muscles of the body.
- Increase the time you hold this position by the number of deep breaths you perform and number of sets.
- Introduce movement of the arms and limbs into the equation.

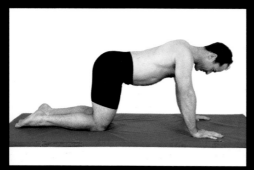

Stomach muscles relaxed

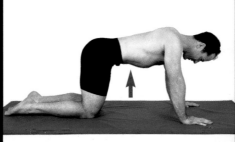

Stomach muscle braced;
Neutral spine maintained; deep breathing constant

Abdominal Bracing Training Focus

Research in lower back injury suggests that the deep stabilizing muscles are best activated at low intensity of around 40% of maximal voluntary contraction (MVC). The reason is the stabilizing muscles are postural muscles that work continuously at low levels of maximal muscle contraction throughout the day. This is easier said than done though as one has to first learn how to activate and control the deeper core muscles. Even though this book is not about recovery from lower back pain, it does have certain merit towards obtaining motor coordination, body awareness and better muscle firing patterns of the deep stabilizers. For maximum benefit one should first learn the anatomy of the body and the roles these muscles play in order to activate, engage or control the MVC intensity. Regular bracing and breathing training will help towards this. Ultimately, one's goal in all exercises is co-activation of the larger trunk muscles in unison with the deeper stabilizing muscles to help stabilize the pelvis and distribute any load across the abdominal musculature in order to avoid stress or overload on the lower back. If at anytime this loads shifts and the lower back becomes stressed or the lumbar region arches or pelvis tilts, the exercise should be stopped. Essentially, all exercises in this book have two key purposes:

1. Strengthen the body whilst also maintaining a strong core position.
2. Strengthening the core is achieved through demands placed on the abdomen-pelvic region whilst performing a number of exercises through different planes of motion – ensuring minimal load on the lower back through effective bracing and breathing (intra-abdominal pressure).

In saying this, at times exercises may require up to 100% MVC in order to achieve this. Then, overtime as one becomes stronger through the core region, especially unloading of the lower back fascia and keeping neutral spine position without arching when performing different exercises, the MVC can be lowered as the muscular framework can effectively brace and hold a similar position at a lower intensity. This means the core is effectively working together.

Bracing of the core therefore needs to be performed in a number of different positions, both statically as well as whilst performing a number of different loaded strength exercises, as different MVC will be required due to the gravitational forces placed on the body:

1. Sitting
2. Kneeling
3. Standing
4. Lying on stomach
5. Lying on side
6. Lying on back
7. Resting on hands horizontally (push-up) and vertically (handstand)

As you increase your body awareness, new abdominal bracing challenges are applied through movement of the arms and legs including a series of low level strength to high intensity plyometric push-up drills performed in a prone position as well as the new cavity-based training approach with exercises performed in a vertical standing position.

Then as bracing, breathing and core strength unite successfully though mastering Phases 1, 2 and 3 within *Core Fitness*, this essential body awareness will allow for Core-in-Motion Method™ (CIMM) Phase 4 development principles to be applied successfully.

Example 2: 4-Point Abdominal Brace Exercise Progression

As an extension to the demands placed on the abdominal brace and breathing pattern as shown in the 4-Point Abdominal Bracing Drill, the 4-Point Coordination Drill raising the opposite arm to leg is applied to further challenge this brace and breath position. Such drills are applied in part 3 of this section through push-ups drills. See section 3 or 4 for similar exercises progressions.

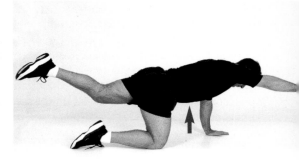

Example 3: Bracing in Motion – Strength Training Exercise

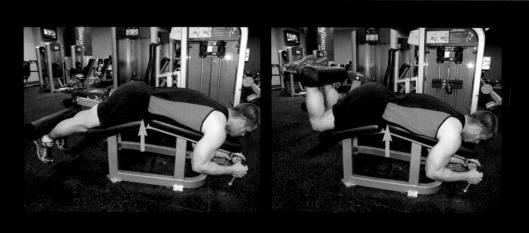

Lie on machine and brace abdominals   Perform leg curl drill

Maintain abdominal brace and neutral spine position. To do this, it may initially require you to lighten the load to avoid arching of the lower back and build specific abdominal bracing endurance and movement synergy with your breathing. As per the 3B's Principle™, with every breath out re-adjust abdominal brace tension to ensure correct body position.

2. Breath

Whilst the abdominal brace focuses on strengthening of the abdomino-pelvic cavity, the development of the thoracic cavity, housing the heart and lungs and linked by the diaphragm, can be also be improved through controlled breathing practices. This principle of deep controlled breathing is the meditational approach that will help enhance lung capacity and oxygen exchange whilst enhancing body awareness and muscle control. The method focuses on continual deep breathing at all times whilst exercising with a particular emphasis on further contraction of the abdominal muscles when breathing out. This insures that a mental focus is maintained until the exercise is completed whilst minimizing the risk of overloading the lower back region when aiming to increase core strength by applying a collective muscle synergy to exercising.

In foundation and core strength training, you **breathe out** when you exert a force – such as rising up from a squat position. You then **breathe in** with recovery – such as lowering the body and bending the legs in a controlled manner when performing a squat. Breathing should remain constant throughout each exercise. In the case of static holding positions such as the Front Support Exercise example we now combine bracing and breathing whilst holding good body position over a set period of time.

Example 4: Front Support Holds in Static Position

The following challenges are designed to build static endurance in a fixed position focused on one's ability to hold a strong abdominal brace and pelvic position to avoid any stress on the lower back. Hence, if at any time the brace is lost or lower back starts to arch, the exercise is stopped.

Instruction
- Start in front support position on hands and toes ensuring eye line is forward of fingers and abdominal muscles are braced.
- Apply a variety of different challenge levels as illustrated.
- Hold strong body position and abdominal brace as you continue to breathe deeply for a set period of time (e. g. up to 60 seconds or more until loss of form).

Note
- Regular small body readjustments are required to maintain good body alignment in all exercises.
- These challenges progress onto push-up drills in motion using the chest and arms to help build core strength in movement as described on pages 90-96.

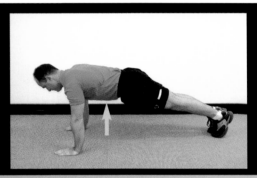

Level 1 – Low intensity

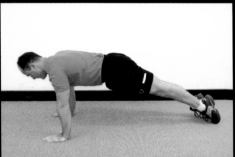

Level 2 – Medium intensity – On point of toes leaning slightly forwards

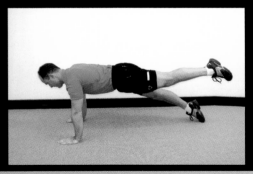

Level 3 – High intensity
Raise one leg whilst maintaining a streamline body position

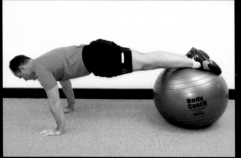

Level 4 (unstable surface) High intensity
Note: Further increase the intensity by raising one leg off ball and keeping pelvis square

3. Body Position

To round out the 3B's Principle™, the third B' relates to one's ability to hold a good body position and technique with each exercise at all times. In all exercises, ensure good head and neck, spine and pelvic alignment is maintained at all times with the rest of the body. The overall focus of each exercise should therefore be on quality of the movement until the exercise is completed.

The 3B's Principle™ - Abdominal bracing and breathing combinations in line with maintaining a good body position at all times should be utilized as a reference point prior to starting and applied whilst undertaking and performing each movement repetition or set.

3. Abdominal Brace Challenge

Horizontal (Cavity) Challenge

In step 3, the abdominal muscle brace can be challenged in a number of ways. In this instance, we use a horizontal (cavity) challenge - push-up exercise - that can include both short and long lever exercise progressions.

Why the push-up is such as a good exercise choice relates to the gravitational force challenge on the body's core. For example, when holding a front support position on the hands and feet, there is a natural inclination for the mid body region wanting to collapse through the core (middle of body being unsupported), placing a tremendous load upon the lower back region.

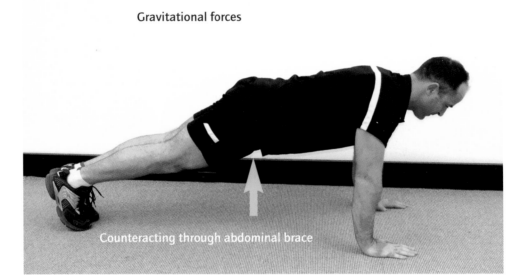

Gravitational forces

Counteracting through abdominal brace

To counteract these gravitational forces (as well as muscle weakness in some athletes), the co-contraction of the trunk muscles with deep stabilizing muscles obtained through an effective abdominal brace helps establish essential intra-abdominal pressure reducing the stress placed on the lower back region by distributing the load across the supporting structures of abdominopelvic cavity whilst performing the push-up exercise.

The crucial point here in core strength training is focused on maintaining this abdominal brace at all times until the repetitions are completed. During this period, if any loss of form or posture occurs, the exercise should be stopped and rest applied before attempting again. This is because, if at any time the abdominal brace releases, the effect will cause lumbar arching or pelvic tilting which in turn places a tremendous amount of stress on the lumbar region.

Push-up Progression Tips

- In most exercises, one's goal is to maintain a strong core postural position whilst using the arms or legs and completing the set amount of repetitions for the specific exercise.

- Whilst building strength in the chest and arms, the focus is also on improving intra-abdominal cavity endurance through bracing and breathing and holding the core in its correct position for the whole exercise time frame.

- In the exercises that follow, start with a close grip variation with hands directly under shoulders. Only widen handgrip placement once strength endurance has been achieved with close-grip variations over a period of weeks to ensure appropriate triceps strength for better shoulder girdle and hip stability.

- Ensure head and neck alignment is maintained at all times with the rest of the body for the development of good posture.

- Ensure neutral spine position is maintained from strong abdominal brace to avoid lower back sagging.

- Start with short lever exercise (on knees) before progressing to long lever (on toes) in order to allow the lower back to adjust to the demands.

- The goal is to progressively improve time performing a set of push-ups (i.e. 20, 40 or 60 seconds continuous) without losing the abdominal brace or technique. This builds essential endurance that enables one to increase the intensity of the push-up exercise from an incline position to on the ground.

- In breathing, breathe out as you exert a force (i.e. push-up or straighten the arms) and breathe in as you recover (i.e. lower the body or bend the arms).

- Additional challenges with the push-up exercise occur through repetition tempo. For instance, 15 repetitions can be performed in both 15 seconds, if 1 second is allowed per repetition before fatigue, or 60 seconds if slowing the exercise down for 2 second count down and 2-second count up for each repetition. This time under tension is important for building upper body and core abdominal bracing endurance and good breathing patterns. Different tempo variations can be applied for good strength gains.

- In Phase 4 we will discuss the next level relating to one's ability to hold a strong core whilst performing dynamic exercises in motion with the Core-in-Motion Method™.

- For more information of cavity-based training, refer to the next step (number 4, page 107).

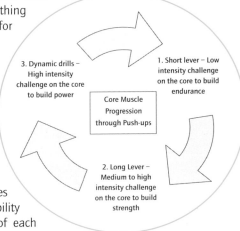

3. Dynamic drills – High intensity challenge on the core to build power

1. Short lever – Low intensity challenge on the core to build endurance

Core Muscle Progression through Push-ups

2. Long Lever – Medium to high intensity challenge on the core to build strength

Outcome: You will gain the ability to hold and maintain a strong core position and deep breathing pattern at all times whilst under load performing various push-ups, and the ability to also adjust the relative MVC to suit the demands of each exercise as you become more efficient in each exercise.

Push-Up Series Progressions: low to high intensity

Modified push-ups allow endurance of the chest, arms, serratus and abdominals to occur through bracing by decreasing the intensity of the push-up exercises through lever length or decline angle of body. As the body angle goes lower to the ground and/or lever length increases, the intensity of the exercise also increases. In saying this, it is important that in the initial development of core strength that modified push-ups are mastered, with the abdominal brace and breathing pattern, and strength endurance obtained (i.e. 30-60 seconds of continuous push-ups without losing form, technique abdominal brace). Start with close-grip position in all three positions – knees and toes – until stronger, before widening grip or performing exercises with hands on ground. Below is a progression of intensity of the abdominal brace required whilst performing a push-up.

1. Kneeling Incline - Short lever, low-intensity push-up exercise for building endurance

Kneel with hands resting on solid foundation such as a bench. Keep arms close against the body when lowering and raising the body with the chest touching the bench. Focus on building muscle endurance whilst maintaining a strong abdominal brace and breathing pattern. A straight line should therefore be maintained from the knees through to the shoulders and head at all times. Breathe in as you lower the body until the chest just touches the bench. Breathe out as you push up to the starting position.

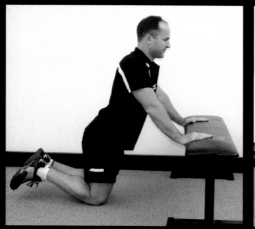
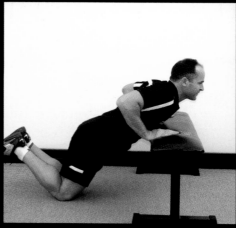

Starting Position **Midpoint**

2. Standing Incline: Long lever, low-intensity push-up exercise on high bench for building endurance

Stand with hands resting forward on solid foundation at approximately waist height, such as a solid table. Exercising at this level can help you achieve good posture and muscle endurance and is a good starting point for the beginner or athletes involved in endurance sports using the upper body such as swimming. The aim is to build muscle endurance of the chest and arms whilst maintaining a strong abdominal brace. Keep arms close against the body when lowering and raising the body with the chest touching the bench. A straight line should therefore be maintained from the heels through to the shoulders and head at all times. Breathe in as you lower the body until the chest just touches the bench. Breathe out as you push up to the starting position.

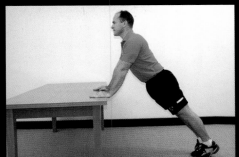
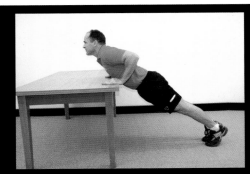

Starting Position **Midpoint**

3. Standing Incline: Long lever, moderate-intensity push-up exercise on low bench

Exercise Description - as per previous exercise (see 2)

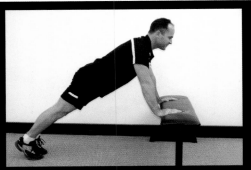
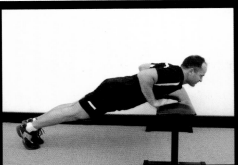

Starting Position **Midpoint**

4.   Kneeling Push-Up

Instruction

- Kneel on floor in a front support position with hands shoulder-width apart and eye line forwards over fingernails.
- Apply 3B's Principle™.
- Breathe in as you lower the body until the chest lowers near the floor.
- Then breathe out as you push-up to the starting position.
- Maintain a tight body from the shoulders to the knee.
- Ensure head and neck alignment is maintained at all times with the rest of the body for the development of good posture.
- Always progress exercise by building muscle endurance with hands and elbows close to body before widening the hand support position. This helps establish triceps strength to support chest strength when widening support position.

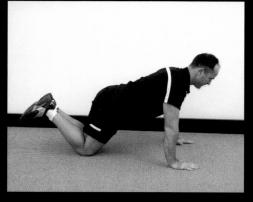
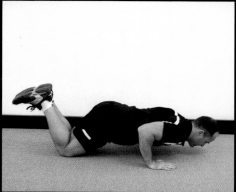

Starting Position   **Midpoint**

5.   Push-Up

Instruction

- Start in a front support position – hands under shoulders, body leaning slightly forward with eye line directly over fingernails and abdominal muscles braced. Apply 3B's Principle™.
- Breathing in, bend at the elbows and slowly lower the body towards the ground with chest over hands.
- Keeping the arms close to the body, breathe out as you straighten the arms.

Note:

- The push-up position itself has a multiple variety of positional changes that can change the MVC required, these include:
  - Close grip push-ups.
  - Shoulder-width push-ups.
  - Wide grip push-ups.
  - Split grip push-ups.
  - Hands resting on object – medicine ball, flat bench or fitness ball.
  - Feet together.
  - Feet wide.
  - One foot raised.
  - Both feet raised on object – flat bench or fitness ball.
  - Plyometric power drills – push-up clap, medicine ball drills, etc.

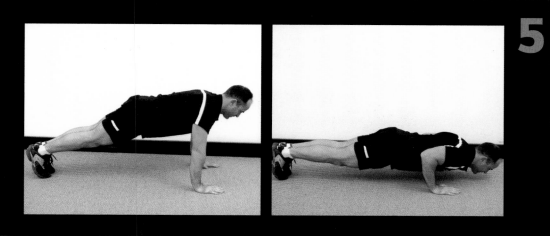

Starting Position   **Midpoint**

6. Medicine Ball Push-Up

Instruction

- Lie on Medicine Ball and place hands on top side with thumbs facing forward – A. Kneeling. B. On Toes.
- Apply 3B's Principle™.
- Breathing out, raise the body up to an extended position.
- Breathe in and lower body.

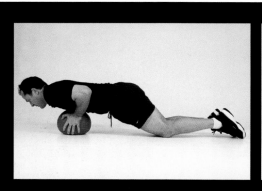

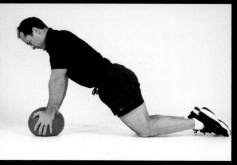

A Starting Position   A Midpoint

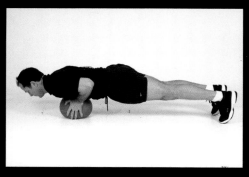

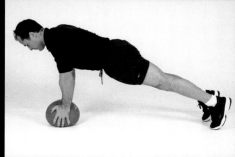

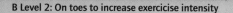

B Level 2: On toes to increase exercicise intensity   B Midpoint

7.   Fitness Ball Push-Up: Hands on Ball

Instruction

- Lie on Fitness Ball and place hands on top side of ball.
- Apply 3B's Principle™.
- Breathing out, raise the body up to an extended position.
- Breathe in and lower body.
- To increase intensity and exercise demand through the core and shoulder regions, raise one foot slightly off the ground when performing push-up.

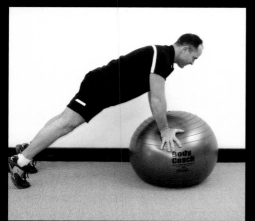
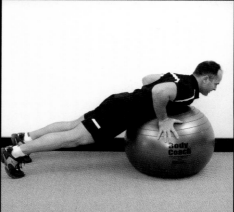

Starting Position   **Midpoint**

8. Fitness Ball Push-Up: Feet on Ball, resting on knuckles

Instruction
- Walk out and place hands in front support position with eye line over fingernails and shins (or feet) resting on ball. Apply 3B's Principle™.
- To reduce wrist stress, clench fist and rest on knuckles (clenched fist).
- Breathing out, raise the body up to an extended position.
- Breathe in and lower body keeping head and shoulders forwards of hands.

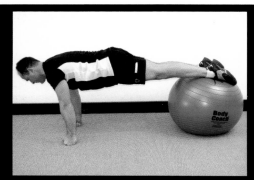 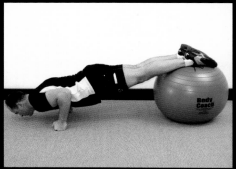

Starting Position   Midpoint

9. Prone Elbow to Front Support

Instruction
- Start in a Front Support position, resting on elbows and forearms with clenched fists on the ground.
- Lean the body forward until eye line is over clenched fists. This ensures strong shoulder position and brace abdominal muscles.
- Apply 3B's Principle™.
- Start by raising up from one forearm onto hand.
- Maintaining strong abdominal brace, rise up onto other hand into a Front Support raised position – hands and toes.
- Reverse sequence and lower back to forearms.

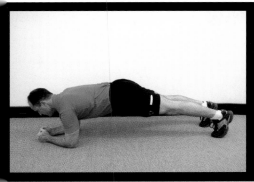

1b. Start

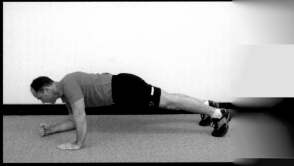

2. Raise onto one hand

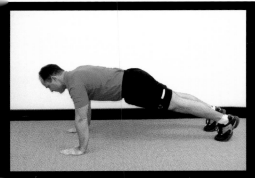

3. Raise on both hands

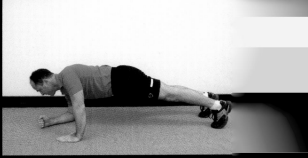

4. Lower onto one forearm and than back to start posi

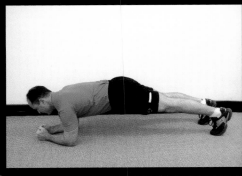

5. Lower onto both forearms

Note

- Perform movement continuously up and down without twisting, tilting or waddling of the hips for set amount of reps or loss of form. This is achieved via a strong abdominal brace at all times, which minimizes any lumbar stress.

- Ensure strong shoulder and abdominal positions throughout exercise.

- Stop the exercise immediately once the core brace is lost or fatigue sets in to avoid any lower back overloading.

10. Front Support Slide - Kneeling

10

Position 1 – Kneeling front support

Position 2 – Extend arms

Position 3 – Arms extend outwards (advanced level only)

- Limit arm range to suit current strength ability.
- Beginners only perform Positions 1 and 2.
- More advanced athletes can advance to Position 3.

Extension to the challenge of the core is achieved by increasing the lever length – varying the angle of the arms and holding this position. The position of the core is held in a banana shape throughout from throughout from knees or feet to the shoulder region.

Instruction
- Start in a four-point kneeling position on hands and knees.
- Lean shoulders and body forward to ensure eye line is forward of fingers. Apply 3B's Principle™.
- Brace abdominal muscles and ensure neutral spine position.
- Hold front support position for 5 seconds then move hands forward 10cm and repeat.
- Maintain these small incremental movements of the hand and holding times until you lose form (i.e. lower back sags) or fatigue sets in with lower back or arms. If so, stop the exercise, rest and recover.

Note
- Limit the arm range extended in relation to one's current shoulder and lat strength ability.
- Beginners only perform Positions 1 and 2. More advanced athletes can advance to Position 3 – holding and then sliding down to the floor to finish exercise.
- This exercise is best learned through the assistance of a coach supporting the hip region.

11.   Front Support Slide – Front Support

Instruction
- Start in a Front Support position on hands with toes pointed.
- Apply 3B's Principle™.
- Hold front support position for up to five seconds then move hands forward 10 cm or so and hold for another five seconds.
- Maintain these small incremental movements of the hand and holding times until you lose form (lower back sags) or fatigue (arms fatigue), then stop, rest and recover.

Note
- Limit the arm range extended in relation to one's current shoulder and lat strength ability.
- Master kneeling exercise shoulder and core strength before attempting the front support drill.
- Ensure head and neck alignment is maintained at all times with the rest of the body for the development of good posture.
- Build stamina by starting with Positions 1 and 2. More advanced athletes can advance to Position 3 – holding and then sliding down to the floor to finish exercise.
- This exercise is best learned through the assistance of a coach supporting the hip region.

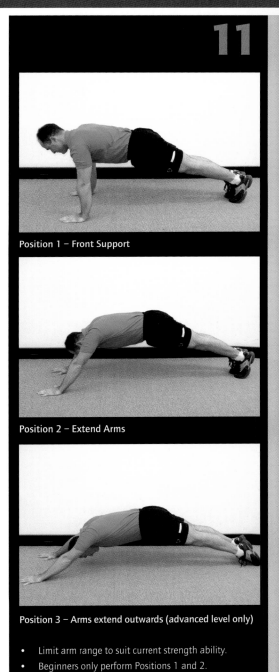

Position 1 – Front Support

Position 2 – Extend Arms

Position 3 – Arms extend outwards (advanced level only)

- Limit arm range to suit current strength ability.
- Beginners only perform Positions 1 and 2.
- More advanced athletes can advance to Position 3.

12.   Seal Walks

Instruction

- Start in front support position on hands.
- Apply 3B's Principle™.
- Point feet and position oneself resting on toenails (socks alone can be worn on carpeted floor for ease of glide).
- Brace abdominal muscles, preferably in reverse dish type position (as per exercise 11).
- Keeping abdominals braced, walk forwards on hands whilst keeping feet together.
- Hands maybe positioned out to the side whilst moving forwards across ground as legs drag (slide) behind you.
- Avoid swinging from the hips or sinking, instead keeping a strong core position with the abdominals braced and legs sliding behind you.
- Maintaining deep breathing at all times.
- Perform over set distance on flat carpeted floor (or on beach across sand).

12

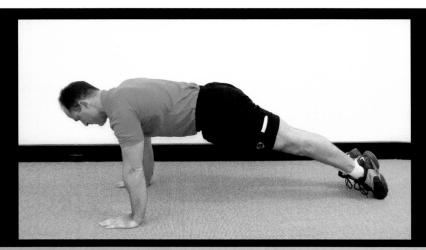

Walk using floor using hands only

13.   Fitness Ball ins-and-outs

Instruction

- Start in front support position with feet on ball and hands on ground.

   Level 1: Shin or ankle (point toes)

   Level 2: Up on toes (as shown)

- Maintaining strong abdominal brace and good body position, roll ball forwards towards chest by bending knees, then outwards to starting position applying 3B's Principle™.

- Continually re-adjust stomach, head and neck alignment and hip position to ensure neutral spinal position is maintained.

- Breathe out when extending legs.

- Breathe in when bringing knees to chest.

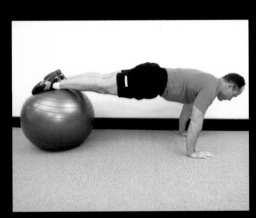 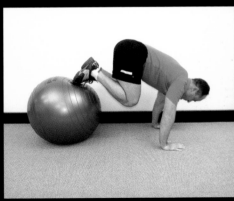

13

Starting Position   **Midpoint**

Bench Press Guidelines – Exercises 14-17

Exercises 1-13 are important in terms of the co-activation between the upper and mid-body as a progressive strengthening continuum. In reaching this point, exercises 14-17 become far more demanding due to the powerful plyometric nature of each exercise which requires specific core body control in line with upper body development through the chest, triceps and shoulder region. The bench press is the most common exercise for developing upper body strength. One's ability to be able to bench press a minimum of their own bodyweight (1:1 ratio) is vital at this point due to the control of eccentric loading demands – for example, push-up clap and landing or pushing hands off medicine ball onto the ground and stopping the body whilst maintaining a strong core. Hence, the following exercises (14-17) and other similar exercises should only be performed under the guidance of a qualified coach – who deems the athlete ready and capable to perform them due to good core strength, muscle control and strength-to-body weight ratio above 1:1.

Instruction
- Lie on your back on flat bench.
- Grip bar evenly slightly wider than shoulder-width apart.
- Maintaining the natural curve of your lower back, brace your abdominal region.
- Breathe in as you lower the barbell towards the midline of your chest.
- Breathe out as you press the barbell to arm's length enforcing a stronger abdominal brace with each lift.
- Maintain a continuous flowing movement at all times until repetitions are completed.
- For more core control, the feet may be raised and legs bent at 90-degrees with abdominals braced.

Note
- The closer the grip on the bar, the more triceps involvement.
- Feet can also be raised, with legs bent in the air for additional abdominal core control required.

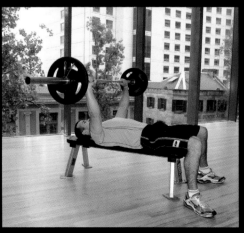 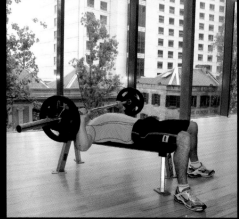

Starting Position   Midpoint

14.   Plyometric Push-ups*

Instruction
- Kneel on ground with hands raised in front of chest.
- Brace abdominal muscles and keep posture strong to avoid arching of the lower back.
- Lean forward and drop to ground keeping knees bent and body straight.
- Absorb forces through eccentric loading of the arms with hands touching ground and arms bending – ensuring the abdominal muscles are braced for core stabilization.
- In one motion upon landing, rapidly push back up concentrically to upright starting position keeping the body tight.

Note
- Maintain strong abdominal brace at all times for core stabilization as quality of movement is paramount over quantity.
- Stop the exercise immediately once the core brace is lost or fatigue sets in, whether after 1 rep or maximum of 10.

Variation
- Eccentric drop and absorb only.
- Eccentric drop and concentric raise.
- Partner holds shoulders and then releases athlete forward for eccentric loading only or eccentric and concentric raise.

* Refer to bench press guidelines page 102

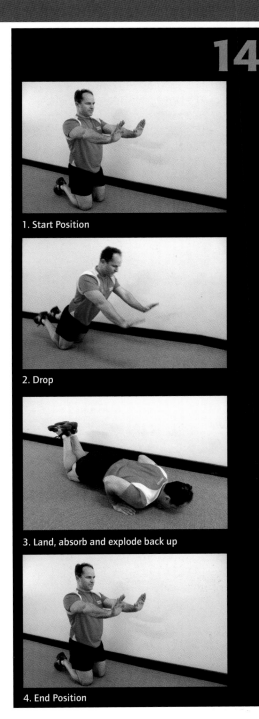

14

1. Start Position

2. Drop

3. Land, absorb and explode back up

4. End Position

15.   Clap Push-ups*

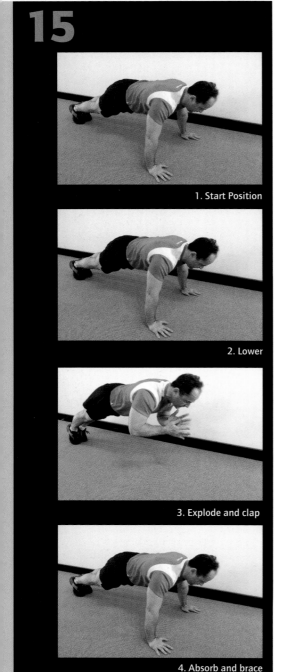

1. Start Position

2. Lower

3. Explode and clap

4. Absorb and brace

Instruction

- Start in a front support position – hands under shoulders, body leaning slightly forward with eye line directly over fingernails and abdominal muscles braced.

- Breathing in, bend at the elbows and slowly lower the body towards the ground with chest over hands.

- Keeping the arms close to the body, breathe out as you explode upwards off the ground bringing hands together to clap, before landing.

- Upon landing, absorb the force by placing hands outside shoulder width and bending the arms – ensuring the abdominal muscles are braced for core stabilization.

Note

- Maintain strong abdominal brace at all times for core stabilization as quality of movement is paramount over quantity.

- Stop the exercise immediately once the core brace is lost or fatigue sets in, whether after 1 rep or maximum of 10.

* Refer to bench press guidelines page 102

16.   Medicine Ball Power Cross*

Instruction

- Begin in push-up position with one hand on medicine ball and elbows bent.
- Brace abdominal muscles and keep posture rigid to avoid arching of the lower back.
- Explode up and across by extending the elbows
- Switch hands on the ball and take opposite hand out to side once again into push-up position.
- Quickly remove hands from the medicine ball and drop down.
- Immediately react and repeat action across to opposite side again.

Note

- Maintain strong abdominal brace at all times for core stabilization as quality of movement is paramount over quantity.
- Stop the exercise immediately once the core brace is lost or fatigue sets in, whether after 1 rep or maximum of 10.

* Refer to bench press guidelines page 102

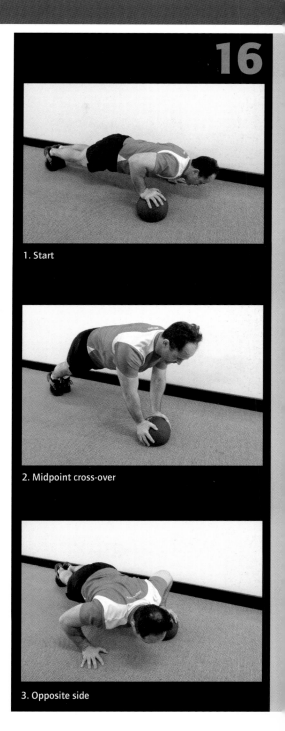

16

1. Start

2. Midpoint cross-over

3. Opposite side

17. Medicine Ball Power Push-ups*

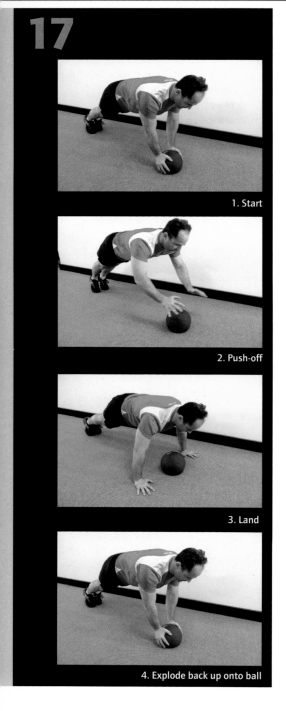

17

1. Start

2. Push-off

3. Land

4. Explode back up onto ball

Instruction

- Begin in push-up position with hands on medicine ball with fingers facing down and thumbs forward.
- Brace abdominal muscles and keep posture rigid to avoid arching of the lower back.
- Quickly remove hands from the medicine ball and drop down.
- Contact the ground with both hands on either side of medicine ball wider than shoulder-width apart.
- Immediately react and push up by extending the elbows, placing hands back on top of the medicine ball.
- Repeat action.

Note

- Maintain strong abdominal brace at all times for core stabilization as quality of movement is paramount over quantity.
- Stop the exercise immediately once the core brace is lost or fatigue sets in, whether after 1 rep or maximum of 10.

* Refer to bench press guidelines page 102

For additional exercises see the following Body Coach Books – Core Strength; Power Training; Abdominal Training

4. Cavity-Based Training Approach

Vertical Position

After progressing through the 17 core challenges in the horizontal front support (push-up) position, in the previous section, we now place the abdominopelvic cavity under stress with a cavity-based training approach focused on exercises primarily performed in a vertical position, on our feet, to imitate the more likely scenario we find in most sporting situations.

The Abdominopelvic cavity can be considered a balloon type structure surrounded by a series of musculoskeletal structures, and upper and lower diaphragm and pelvic floor. The internal cavity itself serves to support and protect the internal organs and lower back (lumbar) region against external loading and stress through intra-abdominal pressure and motor unit stabilization of the deeper muscles when abdominal bracing is activated. Most importantly, this is something we can train to improve through Core-Fitness, Yoga and Pilates-based training.

Gravitational Loading

Sporting movements themselves are very dynamic and explosive in nature and require good core control at all times. To assist towards conditioning these dynamic movements, we introduce the 'squat' exercise. In the squat exercise, a load is placed across the shoulder region (or overhead) whilst the hips, knees and ankles simultaneously bend and lower the load down to a specific leg angle before rising to the upright position. Whilst in most instances one's focus is on lower body strengthening, in this instance we are focusing on the conscious awareness and activation of the abdomino-pelvic cavity with the goal of strengthening the core framework – musculoskeletal, intra-abdominal pressure, pelvic positioning, motor firing and breathing patterns.

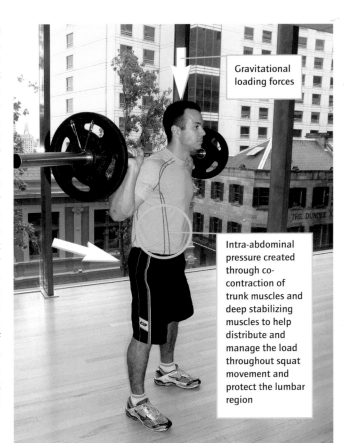

Gravitational loading forces

Intra-abdominal pressure created through co-contraction of trunk muscles and deep stabilizing muscles to help distribute and manage the load throughout squat movement and protect the lumbar region

I like to use this cavity-based training approach in training athletes as it brings attention to increasing one's overall body awareness and muscle control in a vertical position. It also helps them to identify how much contraction and control is required and the specific adjustments that may need to be made whilst in the most efficient postural position before progression onto the Core-in-Motion Method™ (CIMM) in Phase 4. Ultimately, the outcome is focused on improving core strength of the abdominopelvic cavity by increasing the intra-abdominal demand through a series of compound exercises. It also aims to increase the thoracic and abdominopelvic cavity relationship through better breathing, lung capacity, oxygen exchange, body alignment and muscular synergy with movement transfer. Most importantly, the athlete also gains a valuable insight into optimizing lower body strength through core muscle control.

The Wheelbarrow Effect

If you have ever carted a wheelbarrow full of concrete over a set distance for a pour you will have noticed how much core-activation naturally occurs to help stabilize the core region. Yet when the wheelbarrow is empty the likelihood of this occurring is almost non-existent. Why is this so?

When a gravitational load is placed on the abdominopelvic cavity, in this instance – straight arms lifting and holding a heavy load requiring stabilization due to a single wheel moving in a forward motion – intra-abdominal pressure and motor control linked to deep stabilization are switched on naturally requiring a strong abdominal brace in order to perform the activity. At the opposite end of the scale, when there is little or no weight, just an empty wheelbarrow, the demand requires minimal motor recruitment as the sensory and central nervous systems supplies the minimal firing required. Hence, in which instance would the person more likely get injured?

In general, the likelihood of injury will heighten from the fatigue after lifting a number of heavy loads over an

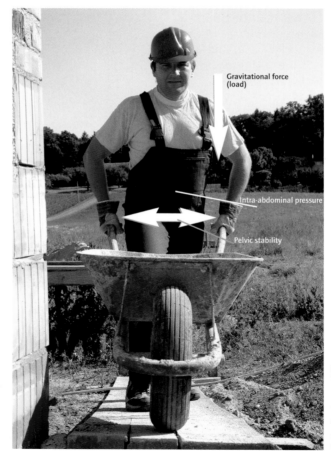

Gravitational force (load)

Intra-abdominal pressure

Pelvic stability

© fotolia, Roman Milert

extended period and returning back with an empty load, where any sharp or sudden movement can overload the supporting structures of the spine due to low level recruitment of the deep stabilizing muscles. When lower back injury does occur, the stabilizing function of the deep stabilizing (multifidus; transversus abdominis) muscles is delayed – I say this from experience. Hence, I'm writing here to you to explain the importance of the implementation of abdominal bracing and breathing through the 3B's Principle™ with each exercise within this book – some automatically activating the core whilst others requiring full core activation. So, even when the exercise may feel easy, this is the time when you want to ensure the core is activated. This way you gain this unique inner body awareness which helps towards improving coordination and timing of the body, making movements that were once demanding more efficient and synergy throughout the body increased as the body works more efficiently.

1.   Body Weight Squat

Co-contraction of trunk muscles and deeper stabilizing muscles of the spine, with little or no load, is vital to install core-control and mind-body relationship. This is a good warm-up exercise prior to lifting or any physical activity along with additional Pre-activity Range of Motion Exercises (PROM) in Phase 1 in establishing vertical core strength.

Instruction
- Stand with feet shoulder-width apart, arms extended forward and parallel with ground. Apply 3B's Principle™.
- Establish foot arch, knee and hip alignment.
- Breathe in; bend the knees and lower body maintaining good body alignment.
- Maintain neutral balance and alignment through ears, shoulder, knees and feet.
- Breathe out and rise upwards to complete one repetition.
- Perform the exercise slow and controlled (i.e. 2 secs up and 2 secs down) focusing on good alignment and body position.

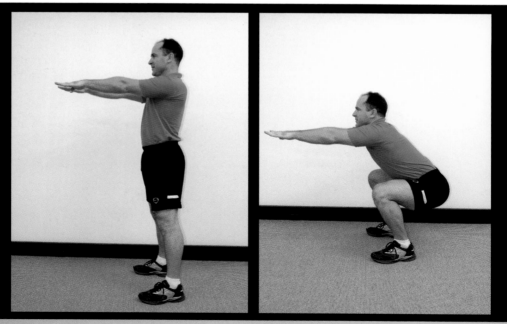

Start   Midpoint –Good Alignment

2.   Medicine Ball Push-Press

As the load increases, so too does one's awareness towards co-contraction of the deep stabilizing and trunk muscles for better movement efficiency and unloading of the lower back and spreading any stress across the core-region itself. This is because your objective is to never feel lower back stress in any exercise.

Instruction
- Stand with feet shoulder-width apart, arms bent holding Medicine Ball against chest.
- Align feet and knees for natural foot arch. Apply 3B's Principle™.
- Breathe in whilst simultaneously bending the hip, knee and ankles and lowering the body towards a 90° degree knee angle.
- Maintain neutral balance through shoulder, knees and feet.
- Breathe out and raise upwards extending the arms overhead.
- Keep abdominals braced, back flat and body long.
- Breathe in as you lower to complete one repetition.

Note
- Ensure proper squat mechanics are maintained.
- Progress to squat with medicine ball release in open area (i.e. field).

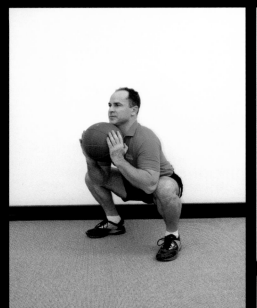
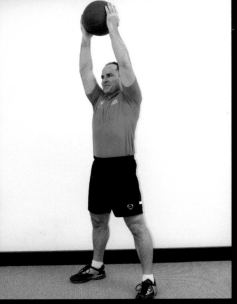

2

Start   Midpoint

3.   Back Squat

As a load is introduced on the shoulders, core-contraction is activated naturally although enhanced through the application of the 3B's Principle™ – which is maintained throughout the entirety of the exercise from start to finish.

Instruction
- Stand with feet shoulder-width apart and bar resting across rear of shoulders with hands slightly wider than shoulder-width apart gripping bar. Apply 3B's Principle™.
- Maintaining the natural curve of your lower back, brace your stomach.
- Breathe in as you slowly bend at your knees, sit back and lower buttocks towards the ground to the appropriate angle – quarter, half or full squat.
- **Note:** Keep your heels on the floor and resist leaning forward from the hips. Maintain ear over shoulder, over hip over ankle – from side position – and knees following the line of the toes.
- Breathe out as you raise body upwards using your legs to starting position.
- Maintain a continuous flowing movement at all times until repetitions are completed.

Note
- This exercise can be performed lowering to a quarter squat, half-squat (90-degree leg angle) or full squat position (advanced athletes only).

3

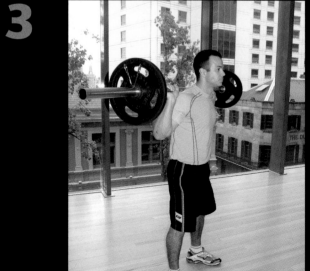

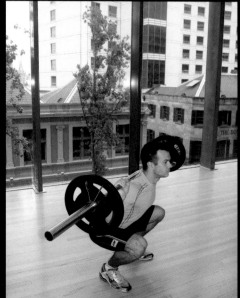

Start   Midpoint

4.   Front Squat

As a load is introduced on the front of the shoulder, core-contraction is activated naturally although enhanced through the application of the 3B's Principle™ – which is maintained throughout the entirety of the exercise from start to finish. It is important that good shoulder flexibility be established to ensure correct hand and arm position whilst resting the bar across the front of the shoulders for ensuring better movement and abdominal cavity control.

Instruction
- Stand with feet shoulder-width apart and bar resting across rear of shoulders with hands slightly wider than shoulder-width apart.
- Maintaining the natural curve of your lower back, brace your stomach.
- Breathe in as you slowly bend at your knees, sit back and lower buttocks towards the ground to appropriate the angle – quarter, half or full squat.
- Breathe out as you raise body upwards using your legs to starting position.
- Maintain a continuous flowing movement at all times until repetitions are completed.

Note
- This exercise can be performed lowering to a quarter squat, half-squat (90-degree leg angle) or full squat position (advanced athletes only). Practice wrist, forearm shoulder and back flexibility regularly to help keep elbows high at all times in order to perform this exercise correctly (see page 31-35).

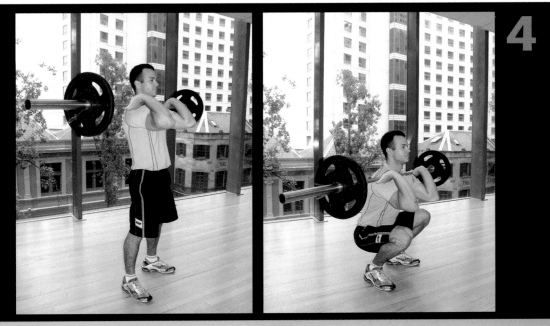

Start   Midpoint

5.   Dead-Lifts

As the angle and load changes you now need to bring your entire focus to movement efficiency and timing ensuring co-contraction throughout the trunk region in line with the 3B's Principle™ to ensure the lower back is protected and any stress through this region is distributed effectively.

Instruction
- With barbell resting on ground, lower body into start position with feet slightly angled out approximately shoulder-width apart; shins close to the bar; knees and hip bent and arms extended holding bar slightly wider than shoulder-width outside knee alignment. Think hips, higher than knees but lower than shoulders – whilst arms are straight and extended down. Apply 3B's Principle™.
- Maintaining the natural curve of your lower back, brace your stomach.
- Breathe out as you simultaneously rise - straightening knees and hip region - into an upright standing position. During the lift, the bar will travel as close to the leg and shins as possible.
- **Note:** If the hips rise before the shoulders, it means you are using your back rather than your legs. If so, reduce weight and perform exercise correctly before progressing. In this movement, most of the weight will be on the heels of the feet to help facilitate maximal contribution of the glutes and hamstrings.
- Breathe in as you raise back up to starting position reversing the lowering position simultaneously.

Note
- Quite often as the weight gets heavier an alternate grip is used with one palm of hand facing towards you and the other palm facing away. Alternatively wrist straps are often used with the conventional grip.
- A more advanced version of the dead-lift for advanced athletes in the straight leg (Romanian) dead-lift. Use only under direct supervision.

5

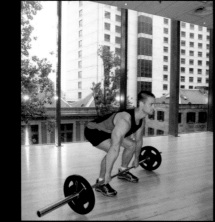

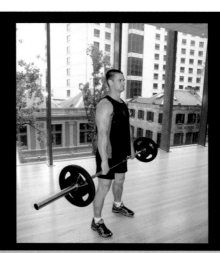

Start Position   Midpoint

6.   Lunge (1): Alternate Leg and Angles

Co-contraction of trunk muscles and deeper stabilizing muscles of the spine, with little or no load, is vital to install core-control and mind-body relationship. This is a good warm-up exercise prior to lifting or any physical activity along with additional Pre-activity Range of Motion Exercises (PROM) in Phase 1 especially in terms of pelvic positioning and establishing vertical core strength.

Instruction
*   Stand tall, feet together hands on hips. Apply 3B's Principle™.
*   Breathing in, step forward (lunge) and slowly lower your body by bending your knees – keeping your knees aligned over your toes.
*   As your rear knee reaches approximately 5 cm from the ground, breathe out through pursed lips, activating a strong abdominal brace, and push back up to the upright starting position.
*   Repeat desired repetitions on one leg, and then the other.
*   In addition, lunge forwards, diagonally, sideways and backwards – see Stage 2: for Lunge Test training example (page 33-54).

Note
*   Keep tall through the chest and aim to make movement flow efficiently.
*   Keep knee aligned over toe.
*   Maintain a strong pelvic position parallel to ground at all times without letting the pelvis tilt or lower on one side with all exercises.

Variation
*   **1. Walking Lunge:** Lunge forward in a continuous fluent walking lunge motion, keeping hips square, abdominals braced, chest tall and body upright.
*   **2. Stair Walking:** Lunge upstairs between 2-4 steps at a time depending on your limb length, keeping hips square, body upright and abdominals braced.

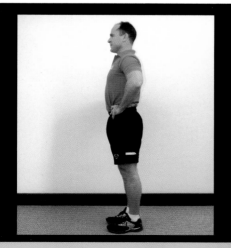 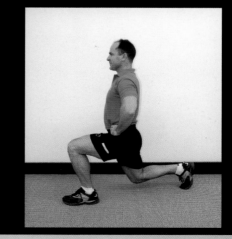

6

Start Position   Midpoint

7.   Lunge (2): Weighted Stationary

With the load distributed across the shoulders, it is vital that the abdominals be drawn in and braced to ensure good pelvic alignment at all times during this exercise when performing in a stationary position with both legs.

Instruction
- Stand with your back straight, barbell across back of shoulders in forward lunge position with hands wider than shoulder-width apart – body raised.
- Maintaining the natural curve of your lower back, brace your stomach.
- Check that both your feet are facing forwards. Apply 3B's Principle™.
- Breathe in as you lower rear knee towards the ground, though never touching.
- Breathe out and rise up.
- Ensure hips remain square at all times.
- Maintain a continuous flowing movement at all times until repetitions are completed, avoiding any arching of the lower back.
- Repeat drill with opposite leg forward.

Note
- This exercise can also be performed with arms extended overhead as shown on page 118.

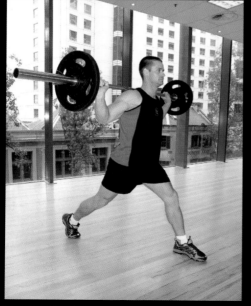
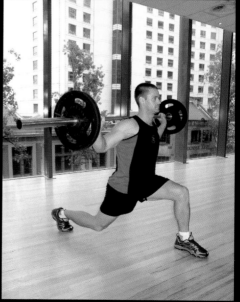

Start   Midpoint

8.   Lunge (3): Alternate Leg

As the exercise demand is increased from a stationary position to a movement lunge forward and back, the core region needs to ensure pelvic alignment is maintained to avoid forward anterior tilt and/or lateral tilt from poor muscle control. Always reduce the weight if this occurs and build the appropriate strength and muscle control before moving forwards.

Instruction
- Stand with your back straight, feet together, barbell across rear of shoulders with hands wider than shoulder width gripping bar.
- Maintaining the natural curve of your lower back, brace your stomach.
- Breathe in as you take a lunge step forward with your left foot.
- Check that your feet are facing forward and your right knee is positioned on the midline of your toe and heel, lowering your right knee towards the ground, though never touching.
- Breathe out as you push firmly back drawing your left leg back and stand upright. Push from your heel keeping your body tight.
- Ensure hips remain square at all times.
- Repeat lunging forward with opposite leg.
- Maintain a continuous flowing movement at all times until repetitions are completed.

Note
- This exercise can also be performed with arms extended overhead as well as continually moving forwards performing a walking lunge.

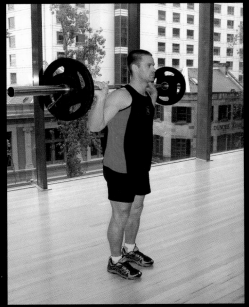
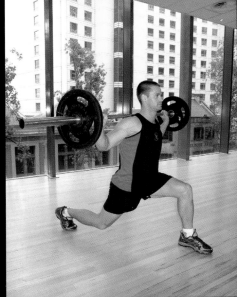

Start   Midpoint

9. Lunge (4): Overhead Stationary Lunge

As the arms are extended overhead and the legs split apart, one's ability to hold the core in its correct position whilst performing this exercise is heightened. Hence, start with little or no weight first and practice to ensure co-contraction and 3B's Principle™ is applied at all times through one's full range of motion and prior to adding any weight to the bar.

Instruction
- Stand tall in forward lunge position with arms extended overhead holding weighted barbell. Apply 3B's Principle™.
- Maintaining the natural curve of your lower back, brace your abdominal muscles and ensure good pelvic alignment at all times.
- Breathe in and lower rear knee towards ground – keeping pelvis square and avoiding arching of the lower back at all times.
- Breathe out and rise up again.
- Maintain a continuous flowing movement at all times until repetitions completed ensuring hips remain square.
- This is an advanced exercise for elite athletes only. Stop the exercise immediately once the core brace is lost or fatigue sets in.
- Always use a spotter or coach for support.
- Repeat set with opposite leg.

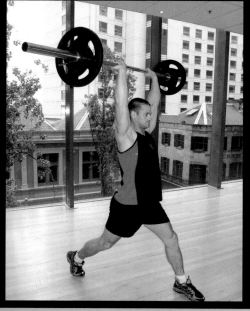

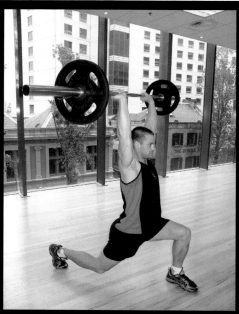

Start   Midpoint

10.   Standing Military Press

As you push any weight overhead, ensure the co-contraction of the trunk muscles remain to avoid any lower back arching. Correct bracing through the application of the 3B's Principle™ brings focus to the exercise at hand and strengthening of the abdominopelvic cavity.

Instruction
- Stand tall resting barbell across front of shoulders with elbows high and hands shoulder-width apart. Apply 3B's Principle™.
- Maintaining the natural curve of your lower back, brace your stomach.
- Breathe out as you press the barbell to arm's length overhead.
- Breathe in as you lower the barbell in front of body to shoulder height.
- Maintain a continuous flowing movement at all times until repetitions are completed, resisting any arching of the lower back.

Note
- This exercise can also be performed standing in a lunge position. It also progresses onto a push-press exercise using the legs to drive the bar up overhead.
- Alternatively, the bar can start resting behind the neck on the shoulders or using dumbbells for more variation and control.

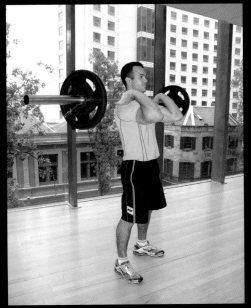 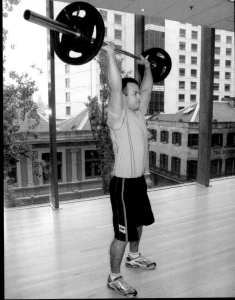

10

Start   Midpoint

11. Barbell Push Press – Front

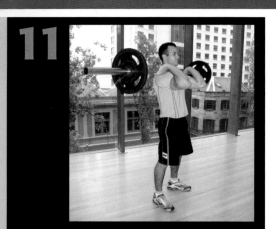

1. Start

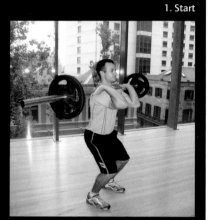

2. Dip

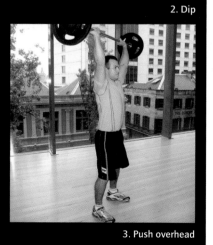

3. Push overhead

Instruction

- Start with barbell resting on front of shoulders and support by hands at shoulder-width – keeping the elbows high.
- Breathing in, drop the hips slightly as part of the initial movement before breathing out whilst exploding up and bracing the abdominal region ensuring hips remain square.
- The objective is to aggressively push up on the bar after driving the legs.
- Unlike the standing military press, the athlete should not be using the arms to drive the weight, but instead use the hips, legs and core.
- The Push Press exercise is used to improve jerk drive through the use of the legs as the primary mover and core region as the stabilizer between upper and lower body.
- To lower the weight, drop it forward onto the platform if heavy. If a lighter weight is used, dip under the bar when lowering back onto front of shoulders.
- Stop the exercise immediately once the core brace is lost or fatigue sets in.

12.   Bent Over Row

As the angle and load changes, you now need to bring your entire focus to movement efficiency and timing ensuring co-contraction throughout the trunk region in line with the 3B's Principle™.

Instruction
- Stand tall gripping barbell at arm's length with hands and feet shoulder-width apart - resting bar across thighs.
- Apply 3B's Principle™.
- Bend at the knees and hip region and slightly lean forwards with bar extending down below shoulders.
- Maintaining the natural curve of your lower back, brace your stomach.
- Tuck your upper arms into your body, whilst keeping your wrists straight.
- Breathe out as you pull bar straight up to your chest keeping elbows close to the body.
- Breathe in as you lower the bar.
- Maintain a continuous flowing movement at all times until repetitions completed, resisting any arching of the lower back.
- Keep your head, neck and back in neutral position at all times.

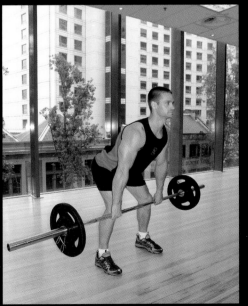 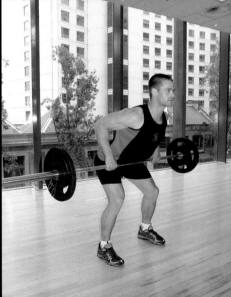

12

Start   Midpoint

Phase 4:
Core-in-Motion Method™ (CIMM)

Objective:

- Build core stamina, strength and endurance – in motion – by utilizing low to high intensity fitness and power based training drills.

- Establish a functional core strength foundation that enables one to maintain good posture at all times towards improving athletic performance.

Phase 4: Core-in-Motion Method™ (CIMM)

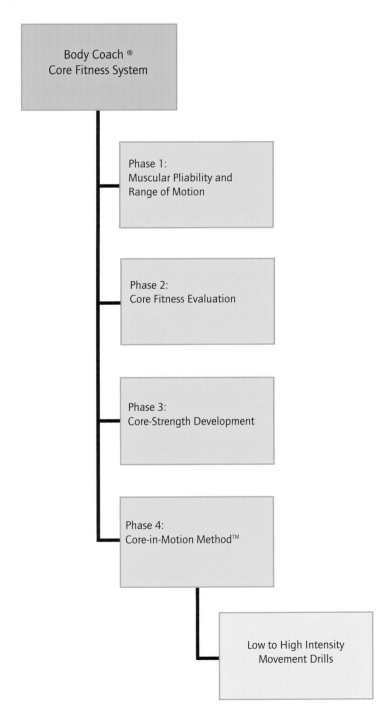

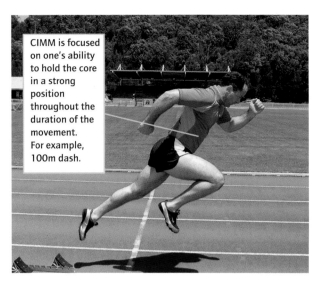

CIMM is focused on one's ability to hold the core in a strong position throughout the duration of the movement. For example, 100m dash.

Upon reaching Phase 4, you will have already grasped the importance of the first three phases in this program. Any athlete involved in sports requires a strong core in order to participate at their optimal level over an extended period of time. The Core-in-Motion Method™ (CIMM) is an extension to the Cavity-Based Training Approach in that the training effort is now combined with physical fitness for building core-stamina in highly demanding and more sports specific positions or motions. In saying this, Phase 1 should always precede Phase 4 as an effective warm-up.

The focus upon which the CIMM will improve your performance will be based on the type of sport you are involved in. Most team field sports, for instance, involve two halves or four quarters of high intensity intermittent exercise, as opposed to continuous prolonged exercise such as that performed by a long distance runner. Individual sports such as tennis, squash, badminton and alike involve games of high intensity bouts followed by periods of recovery between points, games or sets. If you're involved in field events in athletics or Olympic weight lifting, efforts can be highly explosive over very short periods of time, just seconds, with extended recovery before repeating. In track events such as the 100-meter dash a sprinter may only breathe once over the brief 10-second period whilst holding a strong core, whilst a 400m runner requires a strong core for up to 45-50 seconds during the race.

At the opposite end of the scale you find water based sports such as swimming where a 100-meter freestyle swimmer requires good core control through the water for better streamlined body position whilst using the arms and legs for 46-to-52 seconds for the elite male and female athlete respectively, whilst a K1 kayak on the water may take 3-and-a-half minutes to travel 1000-meters whilst maintaining a strong core.

My point being that every sport is unique in terms of fitness, strength, speed, agility, coordination and power requirements. Daily, weekly, monthly and yearly training (periodization) plans are essential to support one's training goals. What core fitness aims to provide you with is an essential platform of core strength over specific periods of time specific to the various sports mentioned above. This is because not all core strength training is performed in the gym. There is another untapped side to core development that I will present to you on the following pages that I've termed the Core-in-Motion Method (CIMM).

Taking Core Fitness to a New Level

As you've learnt in previous phases, core strength is generally performed in a stationary position using one's body weight for general core strengthening as well as various equipment such as fitness balls, medicine balls and strength training equipment alike for the more advanced cavity-based training approach. These phases are necessary for establishing body awareness and a good core strength foundation to build upon.

Now that you've reached Phase 4, the following exercises will assist you in transferring this hard-earned effort into optimal movement efficiency in physical activity and sport by imitating such movements with core-control in mind. For example, with increased loads placed on the shoulders when performing a squat exercise, this will help prepare you for more dynamic movements such as jumping or hopping and landing by conditioning the core cavity region in line with the muscles of the lower body, so it remains braced throughout more dynamic movements ensuring optimal body positioning for achieving increased performance gains.

"....the ability of an athlete to hold a strong abdominal brace and abdominopelvic cavity position when performing a dynamic drill, activity or movement pattern is the key element often overlooked in speed, power and plyometric training – which we aim to address here with the Core-in-Motion Method™ (CIMM). "

In saying this, the ability of an athlete to hold a strong abdominal brace and abdominopelvic cavity position when performing a dynamic drill, activity or movement pattern is the key element often overlooked in speed, power and plyometric training – which we aim to address here through the Core-in-Motion Method™ (CIMM).

With the implementation of the Core-in-Motion Method™ (CIMM) the objective of plyometric training, for instance, will make sense. This is because apart from strengthening the muscles of the arms and legs for more powerful drive, the ability to control and drive this powerful movement is also achieved through one's intra-abdominal cavity bracing ability and ongoing breathing patterns. With the abdominals effectively braced, better movement efficiency will occur because the body is better aligned over extended periods of time with better firing patterns.

The CIMM approach now allows athletes and coaches to train with more clarity and focus by enabling them to gauge one's posture and abdominal brace when performing an exercise. So, ultimately when one's abdominal brace starts to release or the pelvis starts lose its correct positioning causing poor form - the exercise should be stopped. With this in mind, repetitions for powerful exercises can often be focused on one's ability to hold the correct position for a set amount of time. Obviously the more force or energy (intensity) put into an exercise effort will also have an effect on the type of training and exercises performed and for how long. Overall, the Core-in-Motion Method™ (CIMM) aims to bring one's focus to include the development of intra-abdominal bracing and breathing control as a feature of training drills over longer periods when performing movement based dynamic exercises essential for each sport. This includes applying sports specific bracing and breathing techniques whilst in motion over timed intervals or set distances in running, cycling, swimming, rowing and so forth or on various fitness machines.

Success Story

I first applied the Core-in-Motion Method™ with Commonwealth Paralympic (S8) swimming champion Ben Austin leading into the Athens Games – both in and out of the water. A progressive core strength approach was utilized that included coordination drills, resistance drills, water-based drills as well as low impact stationary spin bike repeat training efforts building up to specific water based race times maintaining core pelvic positioning and bracing and breathing techniques with the legs at high velocity. As muscle coordination began to improve in line with effective bracing and breathing techniques the leg turnover on the spin bike he was able to achieve whilst maintaining a strong core position and effective breathing pattern allowed him to train more efficiently in the water, leading to winning 2 gold, 3 silver and 1 bronze medal in Athens including world records in 100m freestyle and 100m butterfly.

Putting CIMM into Action

CIMM includes a progression of low intensity movement based drills towards high intensity powerful plyometric drills and speed based training. Each drill or training effort involve functional movement patterns that challenge one's core position, abdominal brace and breathing mechanism in motion including:

- Rotational
- Lateral
- Skipping
- Low intensity Plyometric Drills
- High Intensity Plyometric Drills
- Agility
- Resisted
- Cycling
- Speed Based
- In the Water

For additional CIMM exercises also see the following books:
- The Body Coach: Power Training Basics
- The Body Coach: Functional Fitness
- The Body Coach: Core Strength Basics
- The Body Coach: Speed for Sport
- The Body Coach: Strength Training for Men
- The Body Coach: Athletic Abs

1.   Body Dish Rolls

This drill helps improve core control in rotation in a horizontal position

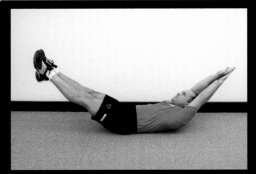

1. Start

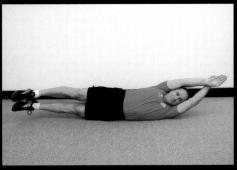

2. Roll to side

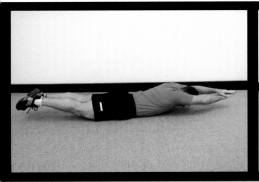

3. Roll onto stomach

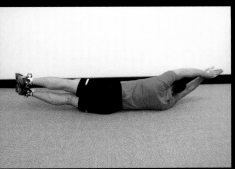

4. Across to opposite side

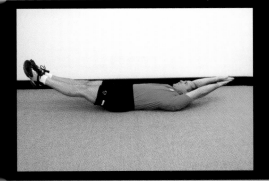

5. Returning to starting position

Instruction

- Rise into dish position, then slowly roll onto side, then stomach maintaining a long extended body position.
- As you roll the body, the legs and arms need to adjust accordingly when rolling onto side then stomach before returning to the first dish position on your back.
- Ensure muscle synergy, speed of movement and body position is maintained.
- Perform single or multiple rolls across a clear floor going to the left and to the right.
- Maintaining a straight line is the athlete's goal.

Exercise Tips

- Use carpeted floor or exercise mats and ensure a clear open space when performing body roll.
- Maintain total muscle control and contraction until drill is completed.
- Maintain 3B's Principle™.

2. Collins Functional Body Rotations™: 180-to-360 Degree Fitness Ball Rotations

This drill helps improve core control in rotation in a horizontal position

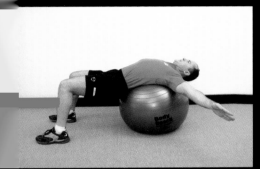

1. Start – Finish

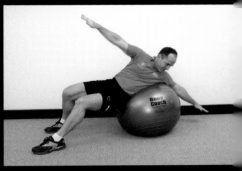

2. Rotation

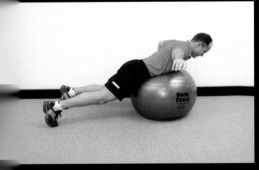

3. Stomach (end of 180-degree)

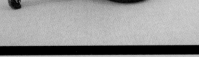

4. Rotate

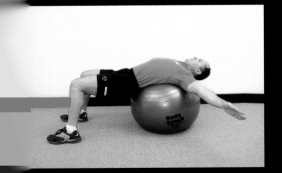

5. End position (360-degree rotation)

Instruction 180-degree Rotation

- Lie on ball at shoulder height across shoulder blades.
- Feet shoulder-width apart, arms extended to the side.
- Keeping arms extended, rotate to the left side, maintaining strong feel with the ball across the chest to maintain ball control.
- Rotating to the left moves the ball across to the right side. As a result, whilst rotating lift the left leg underneath the right as you roll onto your stomach and extend it out to side to control movement.
- Reverse movement by rotating arms and bringing left leg back under to return onto your back.
- Repeat movement three times on the left side and back before repeating rotation on the right side.

Progression

- The next progression relates to performing a 360-degree functional body rotation™ on the fitness ball in control at all times – to the left first and then back to the right side.
- Each rotation should travel in a straight line as this means you are rotating in complete control.
- The speed is controlled at all times through body contact with the ball and correct feet placement in rotation.
- The 360-degree rotation can also be performed over a set distance – i.e. 10-20 meters along a line for guidance.

Note

- This exercise develops muscle coordination between the upper and lower body through the body's core. It requires full concentration and awareness for total muscle activation and control.

3.   Medicine Ball Rotational Thrusts

This drill helps improve core control in rotation in a vertical position

Instruction

- Stand sideways 2-5 meters from solid concrete wall with medicine ball to side of body. Apply 3B's Principle™.
- Rotate arms across the body to release medicine ball across to wall at shoulder height.
- Initially allow ball to bounce before catching to develop concentric strength and coordination on both sides of body.
- As core strength and coordination improves, the loading is increased by throwing against wall and catching on the full in front of the body in a rotational manner.
- In all instances rotate on the balls of the feet whilst keeping the abdominal muscles braced.
- Repeat all drills on both sides of the body for set time or amount of repetitions without fatigue, allowing full recovery between sets.

Variation

- Stand 4-6m from wall; thrust ball and allow to bounce before catching (on both sides of body).
- This exercise may also be performed with a partner.

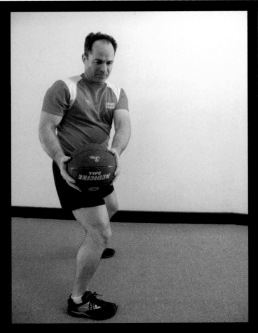 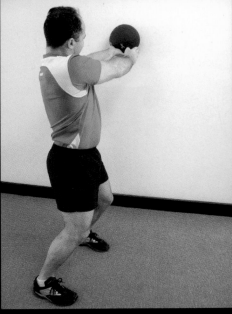

3

4. Side Skips

Lateral side skips help challenge the core in a lateral motion.

Emphasis
- Promote lateral hip stabilizers and core temperature.

Description
- Stand tall, feet together and arms by your side.
- Apply 3B's Principle™.
- Stepping laterally skip leg wide.
- Bring both feet together and then repeat side skip again.
- Continue momentum of lateral skip with feet apart and feet together over set distance.
- Repeat action in opposite direction, leading with the opposite leg.

Variation
- Raise arm parallel to ground and hold whilst feet skip under you.

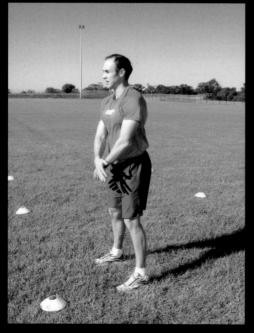 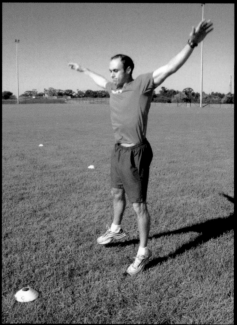

1. Cross arms   2. Side skip and raise arms

5.   Lateral Step–Overs

Lateral step-overs help challenge the core in a lateral motion.

Step 1:   Start with one foot up on the bench and the other foot straddled next to it on the floor.

Push off with the leg that is on the bench and lift your body laterally over so that your opposite foot is on to top of the bench and your other foot is on the ground.

Step 2:   Keeping your back straight and your head up throughout the exercise, lift your body back over laterally across the bench.

Step 3:   Repeat action for desired number of repetitions or length of time. Ensure abdominals are braced throughout the whole exercise to ensure good form at all times – especially pelvic control.

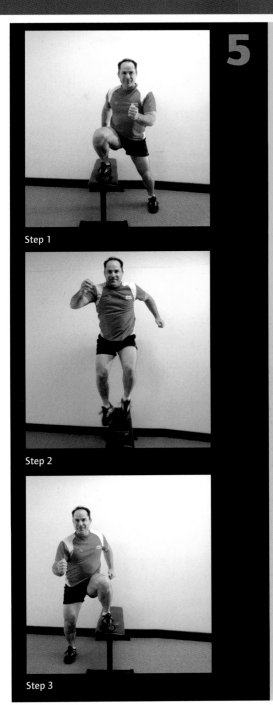

Step 1

Step 2

Step 3

6. Cable Pull-Downs

In this exercise the objective is to focus on squeezing the abdominal muscles inwards each time the arms are pulled down in front of the body. This helps improve upper body and abdominal coordination.

Instruction
- Stand facing lat pull-down or high pulley cable machine.
- Grip bar with palms facing down. Apply 3B's Principle™.
- Activate abdominal brace and focus on deep breathing.
- Breathing out, pull bar down forward of the body towards the hips, maintaining a slight bend in the elbow as you pull down.
- Breathe in and control bar back up to starting point.

Note
- Ensure head and neck alignment is maintained at all times with the rest of the body for the development of good posture.
- This exercise can be performed with a close-grip, natural shoulder-width or wide grip position or lying on back with low-pulley – in a kneeling or standing position.

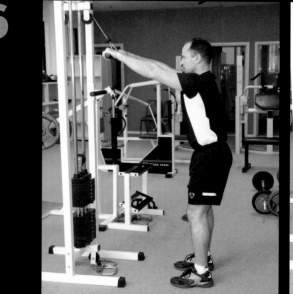 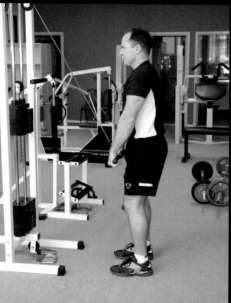

Starting Position   Midpoint

7.   Medicine Ball Power Throw Downs

In extension to exercise 6, the throw down exercise is a powerful movement that includes forming a dish type body position with each jump.

Instruction
- Stand with feet parallel and knees slightly bent.
- Holding medicine ball in hands, extend arms above head.
- Apply 3B's Principle™.
- Brace abdominal muscles and keep posture strong to avoid arching of the lower back.
- Simultaneously jump up as you forcefully thrust medicine ball down in front of body to the ground.
- Land in control by bending the knees to absorb the shock and catch the ball on the first bounce.
- Repeat drill as individual throw down with recovery or repetitive efforts.

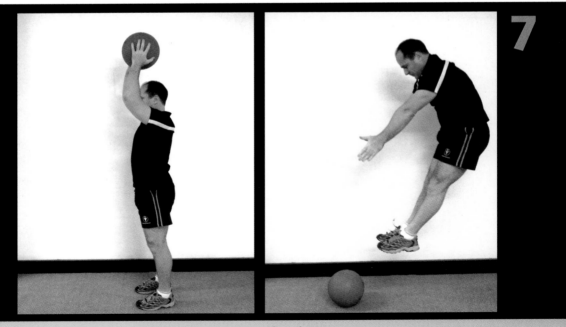

Start   Throw down

8.   Skipping

Skipping is a low level plyometric exercise to assist with abdominal bracing and coordination.

Instruction
- Hold skipping rope in both hands and brace abdominals.
- Apply 3B's Principle™.
- Keep upper arms (elbow to shoulder) close to the body in a relaxed state whilst rotating the hands to jump rope.
- Maintain deep breathing pattern, strong core and relaxed flowing feeling through the shoulders.
- Increase speed and alternate legs as your quality improves keeping the abdominals braced and breathing deep at all times.

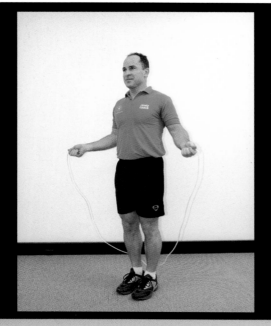

Note

Skipping requires practice. Initially, coordination and timing may not be with you, although, with time and practice you will become very competent in this low intensity plyometric exercise.

9.   Lateral Marker Hops

This drill challenges the core whilst performing hops in a lateral motion on both feet.

Instruction
- Set markers 1-2 meters apart over 10-20 meters.
- Stand behind markers with feet close in a lateral position, legs slightly bent and arms by side. Apply 3B's Principle™.
- Start with counter movement – squat, swing arms backwards.
- Then hop laterally – to the side – up and over marker.
- Bend knees upon landing to absorb shock.
- Upon each landing, take off quickly upward again with the same action.
- Maintain good body posture at all times when jumping and landing as quality of movement is paramount over quantity.
- Rest 5 minutes and repeat action in opposite direction.
- Ensure abdominal brace and pelvic position is maintained at all times.
- Stop exercise if brace releases or form lapses and shorten distance of hop until core strength is improved.

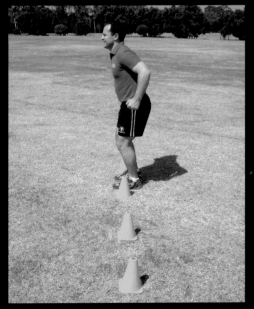 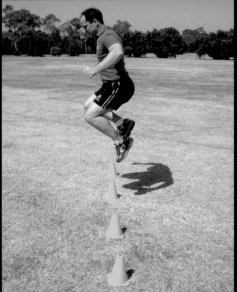

Start   Hop Laterally

10.   Forward Marker Hops

This drill challenges the core whilst performing hops in a forward motion on both feet.

Instruction

- Set markers 1-2 meters apart over 10-20 meters.
- Stand behind markers with feet close, legs slightly bent and arms by side. Apply 3B's Principle™.
- Start with counter movement – squat, swing arms backwards.
- Hop forwards on both feet, up and over markers.
- Upon each landing, take off quickly upward again with the same cycling hop action of the legs – use arms for balance and control.
- Execute the action sequence as rapidly as possible.
- Work on speed of movement, but not at the expense of poor technique.
- Maintain good body posture at all times when jumping and landing as quality of movement is paramount over quantity.
- Ensure abdominal brace and pelvic position is maintained at all times.
- Stop exercise if brace releases or form lapses and shorten distance of hop until core strength is improved.

10

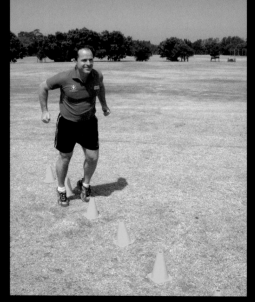

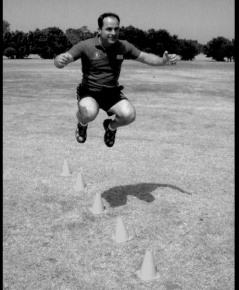

Start

Hop forwards

11. Single-Leg Speed Hop

This drill challenges the core and pelvic position whilst performing a single leg hop in a forward motion.

Instruction

- Stand on left leg next to marker, legs slightly bent and arms by side.
- Apply 3B's Principle™.
- Start with counter movement – squat, swing arms backwards.
- Hop forwards on left leg.
- Upon each landing, take off quickly upward again with the same cycling hop action of the legs – use arms for balance and control.
- Use the multiple-response action of rapid yet fully explosive cyclic action for height and distance.
- Perform single leg hop over 10–20 meters.
- Maintain good body posture and technique at all times when jumping and landing as quality of movement is paramount over quantity.
- Rest 5 minutes and repeat using right leg.
- Ensure abdominal brace and pelvic position is maintained at all times.
- Stop exercise if brace releases or form lapses and shorten distance of hop until core strength is improved.

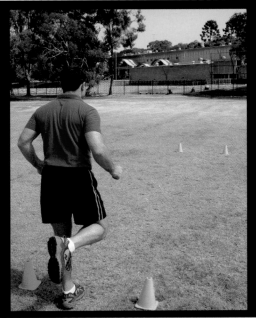
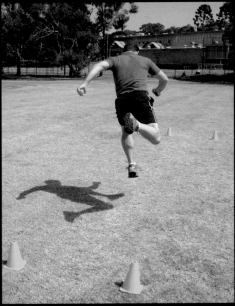

11

Start   Single Leg Hop

12. Single Leg Lateral Marker Hops

This drill challenges the core position whilst performing a single leg hop in a lateral motion.

Instruction (for advanced athletes only)

- Set markers 1-2 meters apart over 10-20 meters.
- Stand behind markers on left leg in a lateral position with right leg slightly bent and arms by side. Apply 3B's Principle™.
- Start with counter movement – squat, swing arms backwards.
- Then hop laterally – to the side – up and over marker.
- Bend knees upon landing to absorb shock.
- Upon each landing, take off quickly upward again with the same action.
- Maintain good body posture at all times when jumping and landing as quality of movement is paramount over quantity.
- Rest 5 minutes and repeat action in opposite direction on right leg.
- Ensure abdominal brace and pelvic position is maintained at all times.
- Stop exercise if brace releases or form lapses and shorten distance of hop until core strength is improved.

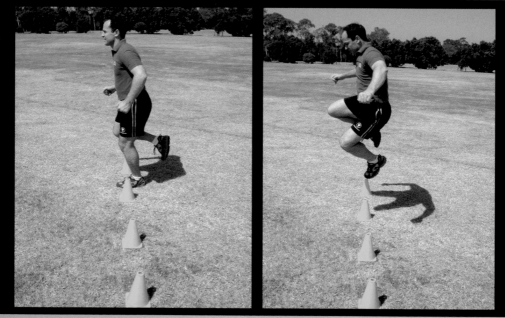

12

Start   Lateral Single Leg Hop

13.   Single Leg Multiple Marker Hops

This drill challenges the core and pelvic position whilst performing a single leg hop in a forward motion.

Instruction (for advanced athletes only)
- Set markers 1-2 meters apart, or as required by athlete over 10 meters.
- Stand behind marker on left leg, with right leg slightly bent and arms by side.
- Apply 3B's Principle™.
- Start with counter movement – squat, swing arms backwards.
- Hop forwards on left leg, up and over marker.
- Upon clearing the first marker, land with full-foot contact and give at the knees and hip – use arms for balance and control.
- Upon each landing, take off quickly upward again with the same cycling hop action of the leg.
- Execute the action sequence as rapidly as possible.
- Work on speed, but not at the expense of poor technique.
- Maintain good body posture at all times when jumping and landing as quality of movement is paramount over quantity.
- Rest 5 minutes and repeat with right leg.
- Stop exercise if brace releases or form lapses and shorten distance of hop until core strength is improved.

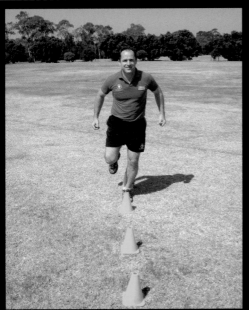

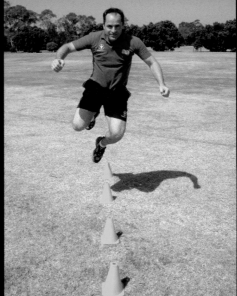

13

Start   Hop

14. Agility Pole Drills

This drill challenges the core and pelvic position whilst performing forward lateral movement, whilst stepping off each foot.

Equipment
- 10 agility poles placed 2-3 meters apart in a straight line.

Description
- Apply 3B's Principle™.
- Lead into agility poles at speed.
- Step across and forward through agility poles as quickly as possible.

Teaching Points
- Work off the balls of the feet as you transfer weight forward and laterally when stepping through agility poles.
- The step force should be equal on both legs.
- Maintain same body height throughout.
- Keep close to agility poles for quicker speed to end point.
- Maintain focus and good body alignment until repetitions completed.

Variation
- Forward swerve with lateral call to sprint (i.e. run forwards through agility poles then on coach's call turn left or right and sprint 10m).
- Lateral running through agility poles.

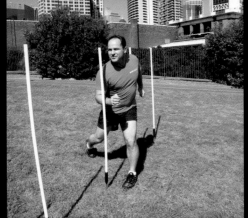

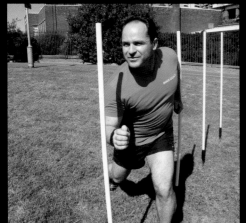

Move rapidly

Stepping in and out of poles

15.   Lateral Quick Steps

This drill challenges the core and pelvic position whilst performing steps forward and backward travelling in a lateral-diagonal motion.

Equipment
- 10 markers, 1-meter apart in a straight line.

Description
- Apply 3B's Principle™.
- Stand side-on and lead into markers laterally at speed.
- Zig-zag legs forwards and backwards laterally through markers.
- Repeat in opposite direction.
- Ensure abdominal brace and pelvic position is maintained at all times.

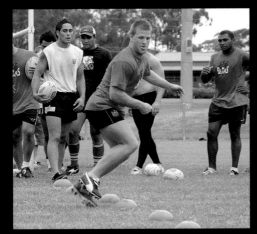 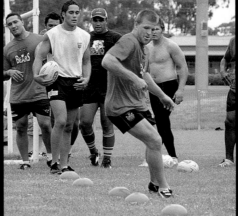

15

Step forward laterally   Step back laterally

16.   High Velocity Stationary Cycling

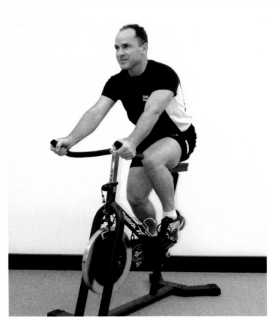

Peddling at high speeds on a stationary bike with varying resistance on the fly-wheel allows you to imitate the leg speed of running or swimming without the stress of impact, especially in relation to running. Various resistances can be added to support both alactic and lactic acid scenarios – through time and fly wheel resistance dependant on one's fitness levels. Whichever the case, one's goal is to ensure the core region is activated and pelvic held in the correct position throughout whilst breathing deeply. Apply similar sprint cycles and recovery period to those on the running track or in the water with light peddling turn-over (less tension on fly wheel) in between reps and sets for aerobic turn-over to assist in any removal or breakdown of lactic acid.

Core Fitness Cycling Sample:
- Warm up: 5 minutes with low resistance focusing on core-control and breathing on stationary bike.
- Session: Perform 12-15 minutes of 30-60 second sprints. Select a level of resistance with each sprint that requires forces and challenges your core at the same time – applying 3B's Principle™.
- If you sprint 30 seconds, recover for 60-90 sec using a light resistance and lower level core-activation and deep breathing patterns. If you sprint for 60 seconds, recover for 90-120 seconds.
- If you like, you can take a 3 minute break after 6 minutes of high intensity effort depending on your condition.
- Warm down: 5 minutes with low level resistance followed by stretching.

17.   Resisted Running: Speed Sled

To assist in a runners speed development, various speed training equipment has been developed that allows similar training resistance effects over shorter periods of time or distances of normal running. These are great training tools for adding variety into a training session and can consist of resisted or overspeed training principles. Always follow manufacturer's guidelines when using this equipment.

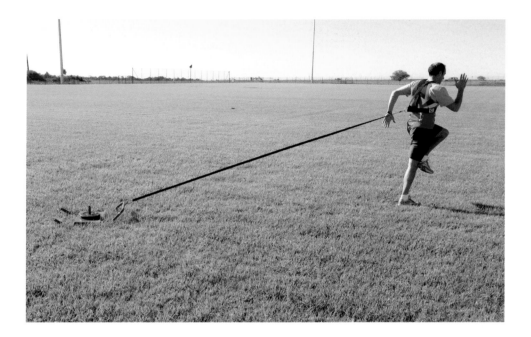

Instruction
- A weight plate is placed onto the speed sled to suit the athletes training requirements. Attach harness around body and secure. Using an open grass area or running track, drive forward in strong running position for repeated efforts over 40 meters with recovery between reps.

18.   Falling Starts

18

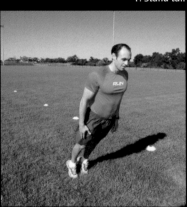

1. Stand tall

2. Raise onto toes and lean forward

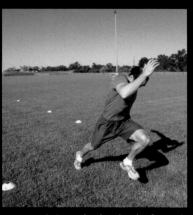

3. React, land and sprint forwards

This drill challenges the core and pelvic position whilst performing a fall into an explosive sprint start motion in a forward direction.

Emphasis
- Improve leg reaction, drive and acceleration.

Description
- Stand tall with feet together and hands by your side.
- Apply 3B's Principle™.
- Lean forward and raise up onto toes until balance is lost.
- React with two quick steps and rapid arm drive followed by short sprint over 10-20m.

Teaching Points
- Look forward with chest held tall and head in neutral position.
- Lean and react with arm drive and two-quick steps.
- Maintain strong core and upright posture.
- Continue good body mechanics for short sprint.

Variation
- After two steps and short sprint, add change of direction – left or right.
- Add decision after short sprint – i.e. dodge, weave or step.
- START and STOP – falling start, sprint 10m and stop. Repeat 4 times.

19.   Stair Drills

Running stairs help develop leg strength and core power.

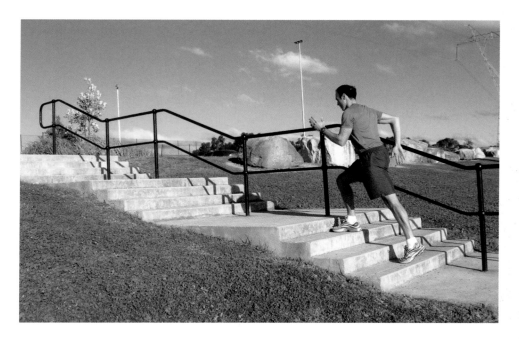

Instruction

- Focus on 6-8 seconds of leg drive up stairs of different inclines including stadium stairs.
- Longer periods will lead to lactic acid build-up, so ensure full recovery periods and light aerobic exercise for breakdown and removal of lactic acid. Both individual stair running and bounds off one leg onto the other over 2 or more stairs at a time may be used depending on one's core stability and power.

Variation

- Walking lunges up stairs, stepping 3-5 stairs whilst keeping hips square, abdominals braced and body leaning forwards helps condition the core for the stair runs.

20. Starts and Accelerations

Instruction

- Place blocks 1 foot length behind line and one foot apart between forward and rear block.
- Put both hands behind line, shoulder-width apart.
- Place both feet into blocks leading with dominant leg.
- Lower rear knee to ground in line with the front foot.
- On 'your marks' call, lean forwards and place hands on line shoulder-width apart – thumbs inwards, fingers pointing out with slight arch between index finger and thumb.
- On 'GO' – explode from line and sprint forwards maintaining a strong core for:
  - 10 meters
  - 20 meters or more

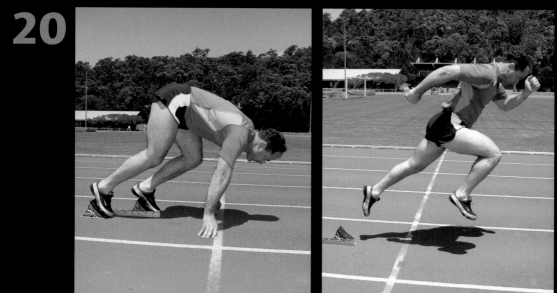

Set   Explode

21. Speed Endurance

Speed endurance will often be sports specific and is related to 80-90% of maximum effort with a brief recovery of up to 3 minutes between reps. Most field sports, for example, require short sprint distances at maximal velocity followed by brief bouts of low intensity effort, walking or being stationary. Hence, interval training is a great way to build one's endurance which helps support maximum velocity efforts and recovery between them. As part of this process, your goal includes being able to hold your core throughout the whole distance running at 80-90% of maximum velocity without loss of form. Below are a few training session examples where this could be used:

- 6 x 80m with 1.5 minutes rest
- 6 x 100m with 2 minutes rest
- 8 x 150m with 2.5 minutes rest
- 6 x 200m with 3 minutes rest

Ultimately, start short and build the distance as one's core becomes stronger. Quality is one's focus, so at times a longer rest period may be required or specific reps and sets be adjusted or split into two groups (eg. 2 x 4 x 150m with 5 minutes rest between sets).

22.   Pure Speed

Pure Speed relates to running at maximum speed over short distances – usually involving up to 6 seconds at maximum intensity in training. For example:

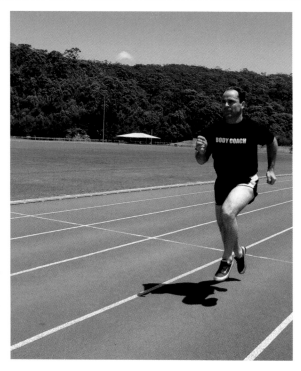

- **Up to 6 seconds maximum effort:** 30-40m or up to 60m from a standing start, Flying 20-30m runs off a 25m build-up.

- **Ins & Outs:** 25m acceleration distance followed by 10m at maximum effort holding one's breath and strong core running into a 20m zone at high cadence with less effort where you breathe out leading into the final 10m zone for another maximal effort with breath held once again before ease out of the sprint, but ensuring the core is held tightly at all times until stopping.

In either example, one's goal is to keep the core region braced and pelvis square at all times during the distance or time right through to the point of stopping. This ensures you are applying the Core-in-Motion Method™ (CIMM).

23.   In the Water

Core fitness can also be developed in the water by maintaining focus on pelvic position and core muscle control with each stroke and breath.

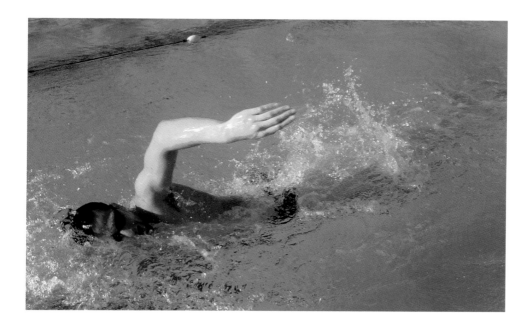

General Core Fitness Session
Core Option 1: Apply 3B's Principle™.
*   100m-400m warm-up (depending on swimming ability)
*   6 x 50m:
    *   2 x 50 m with 30 seconds rest after each
    *   2 x 50 m with 20 seconds rest after each
    *   2 x 50 m with 15 seconds rest after each
*   3 x 100m

Perform each of these 100s with 60 seconds of rest after each. Try to drop 2 seconds from each 100 repeat. This is a great way to learn to pace yourself and build essential core fitness through abdominal control.

200m-400m cool down (relaxed swimming, focusing on breathing and core control).

Core Option 2: Apply 3B's Principle™.

- 100m-400m warm up (depending on swimming ability).
- Using a kickboard - kick 1 x 50m going hard then 1 x 50m going at 70% pace.
  Repeat x 3.; take 60 seconds rest after each 100m.
- Swim 6 x 50 with laps 1, 3 & 6 as hard as you can go focusing on core control and deep breathing at all times; and 2, 4 & 5 nice and easy. Take 20 seconds rest after the easy ones and 35 seconds rest after the harder efforts.
- Swim an easy 100m-200m working on nice long strokes.

Note: If you have ankle flexibility issues or are not from a swimming background, use fins (flippers) for a month as they can help increase your ankle flexibility, allowing you to do swimming drills with ease whilst applying the core-bracing principle, whilst also strengthening the leg muscles for kicking.

Core Fitness Programs

Each sport has a specific need in terms of core-control – some sports are explosive for just a brief period whilst others over an extended period of time. With this in mind, one should always undertake a general preparation period for core strength and body awareness to develop. Then, as core fitness gradually improves, one can apply a more specific approach to the needs of one's sport. core fitness is often seen as supplementary to one's sport, but as you've discovered the importance of the CIMM in training allows you to focus on core strength in motion towards improving one's posture, core fitness and athletic potential.

Determining Repetitions and Sets

In core fitness, determining repetitions and sets will vary depending on the nature of the task or the training outcomes. There are many factors in core fitness training that influence reps and sets including:

- Athlete's training background
- Athlete's ability to hold their core or pelvic position
- Training objective – base work or in-season
- Nature of sport – endurance or power-based
- Type of exercise – Phases 3 & 4
- Time on task
- Time under tension – static position or tempo of exercise (1sec up and 1sec down or 3 sec up and 3 sec down for same amount of reps)
- Speed of movement – individual, slow, explosive, repetitive
- Set distance (i.e. over 10 or 20 meters)

So whilst some drills may utilize 4-8, 8-12 or 12-15 reps for power, strength or endurance respectively, others may best be suited to time on task and will be noted accordingly. In saying this, if at any time one loses their ability to hold their core or pelvic position, the exercise should be stopped and a recovery period undertaken.

Remember, starting out too hard too early can be counterproductive to your development – placing too much stress on already overloaded core framework including muscles, ligaments, tendons and joints or energy systems. Each exercise therefore serves as a test (specific tests in Phase 2). Appropriate core strength can be gauged by the ability of the athlete to maintain a good body position whilst applying the 3B's Principle™.

Recovery or Rest Periods

Allowing 30–180 seconds recovery is recommended between most exercises, if working the same muscle group or the same exercise is being repeated. Recovery is generally based on two key elements:

1. Purpose of your training – low, medium or high intensity (endurance, strength or power based).
2. One's current fitness or strength level.

The longer the recovery period the fresher you will be – choose accordingly.

Training Schedule

In general, athletes should work the whole body at least 3 days per week for general core conditioning for around 30 minutes, with one rest day in between workouts in addition to their normal sports-specific training program. For example: Monday, Wednesday and Friday. This is important as your body recovers and rebuilds whilst resting.

Sample Training Programs

On the following pages are four sample training programs plus a template page for you to design your own specific training program to suit your needs. These programs act only as a guide. Adapt reps and sets and recovery to suit your current level of fitness and training needs. Replace exercises as required (lower or higher intensity). Use template page as you develop in core-fitness.

Core Fitness – General Preparation

Perform Phase 1 warm-up activities prior to all exercises below.

Exercise	Page No.	Reps	Sets	Recovery
1. Body Weight Squat (warm-up)	21	10	1	Nil
2. Back Squat	117	10-12	3	60-90sec
3. Supine Body Dish	62	10sec holds	3	30sec
4. Collins-Lateral Fly™ Series – Long Lever	66	10-20sec	2 each side	Nil
5. Lower Leg Lifts	70	12-15	3	30sec
6. Knee Raises	71	10-15	3	30sec
7. Push-Up (choose level accordingly)	93	10-20	3	60sec
8. Agility Pole Drills	142	10m	5	60sec each rep

Warm down and stretch upon completion of session

Core Fitness – Intermediate

Perform Phase 1 warm-up activities prior to all exercises below

Exercise	Page No.	Reps	Sets	Recovery
1. Lunge (1): Alternate Leg and Angles	115	10	Each leg	Nil
2. Dead-Lifts	114	10-12	3	60-90sec
3. Fitness Ball Push-Up: Hands on Ball	95	10-15	3	60sec
4. Fitness Ball Abdominal Crunch	64	10-20	3-4	60sec
5. Pistons	73	15-30sec	3	60sec
6. Body Dish Rolls	127	10meters	3 each side	15sec
7. Fitness Ball ins-and-outs	101	10-12	3	60sec

Note: Choose 2 x Core-in-Motion Method™ (CIMM) drills to undertake specific to your sports/training needs.

Warm down and stretch upon completion of session

Core Fitness – Advanced

Perform Phase 1 warm-up activities prior to all exercises below.

Exercise	Page No.	Reps	Sets	Recovery
1. Front Squat	113	8-10	3-4	60-90sec
2. Lunge (2): Weighted Stationary	116	8-10	2 each leg	60-90sec
3. Medicine Ball Push-Up	94	10-15	3-4	60sec
4. Medicine Ball Toe Touch	63	10-20	3-4	60sec
5. Medicine Ball Elbow to Knee	69	12	3 each side	60sec
6. Lateral Side Raises	68	10-15	3each side	15sec
7. Hanging Raises (10a)	72	10	3	60sec
8. Plyometric Push-ups	103	6-8	3	120sec

Note: Choose 2 x Core-in-Motion Method™ (CIMM) drills to undertake specific to your sports/training needs Warm down and stretch upon completion of session.

Core Fitness – Elite

Perform Phase 1 warm-up activities prior to all exercises below.

Exercise	Page No.	Reps	Sets	Recovery
1. Lunge (4): Overhead Stationary Lunge	118	8-10	2 each leg	90sec
2. Front Squat	113	8-10	3-5	90sec
3. Lateral Quick Steps	143	10sec	3-5	60sec
4. Medicine Ball Power Push-ups	106	8-10	3-5	120sec
5. Bench Press	102	8-10	3-5	60sec
6. Lateral Side Raises	68	10-15	3 each side	Nil
7. Front Support Slide – Front Support	99	5	1	60sec each rep
8. Hanging Raises (10b)	72	10	3	60sec
Rest 5 minutes and stretch				
9. Pure Speed	150	10x40m	1	90sec walk back
10. Falling Starts	146	5x10m	1	60sec each rep
11. Forward Marker Hops	138	5x10m	1	90sec each rep

Warm down and stretch upon completion of session.

Use the following template to design your own Core Fitness Program

Core Fitness – Template

Perform Phase 1 warm-up activities prior to all exercises below

Exercise	Page No.	Reps	Sets	Recovery

Warm down and stretch upon completion of session

Core Fitness Index

Body Coach® Education and Products

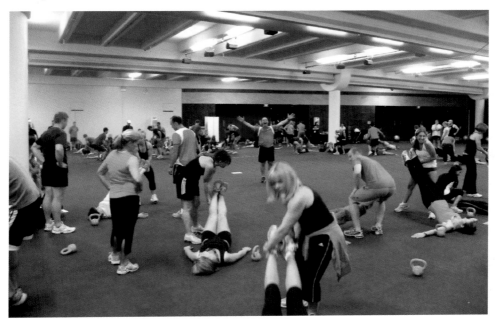

Paul Collins Presenting at International Fitness Conference, Sydney, Australia

Everything you need to know about fitness:

www.thebodycoach.com
www.bodycoach.com.au

Fitness made easy™

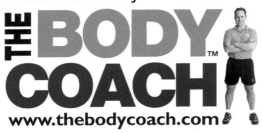

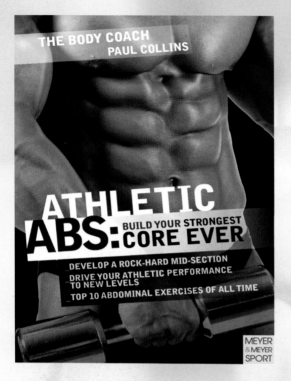

Paul Collins
**Athletic Abs –
Build Your Strongest Core Ever**

Develop core-strength, power and a rock hard mid-section to help drive your athletic performance to a new level. The Body Coach® Paul Collins, Australia's Personal Trainer™, delivers yet another cutting edge training program with *Athletic Abs* by combining a progressive series of abdominal strengthening exercises aimed at improving posture, body awareness, core-strength, motor control and athletic performance.

c.144 pages, full color print
c. 200 color photos
Paperback, 6 1/2" x 9 1/4"
ISBN: 9781841262956
$ 14.95 US/$ 22.95 AUS
£ 9.95 UK/€ 14.95

Paul Collins
Strength Training for Men

Strength Training for Men conditions your body for muscular gains and increasing athletic performance. The Body Coach® Paul Collins, Australia's Personal Trainer™, includes practical, easy-to-follow strength training routines that help guide you through basic lifting techniques to more advanced Olympic-lifting power progressions. Exercises progress from isolated to more complex compound movements that help improve Central Nervous System (CNS) recruitment and muscular coordination. Best of all, each exercise and program is clearly and simply explained. The book is loaded with relevant information for any athlete, coach or trainer at any level.

184 pages, full color print
352 color phot., 20 illustr., 32 charts
Paperback, 6 1/2" x 9 1/4"
ISBN: 9781841262864
$ 14.95 US / $ 22.95 AUS
£ 9.95 UK/€ 14.95

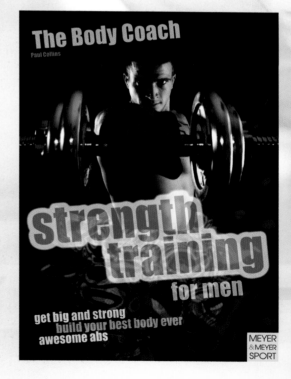

The Sports Publisher

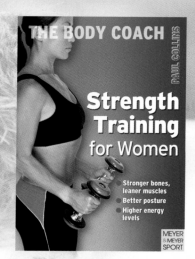

Paul Collins
Strength Training for Women

The combination of strength training, aerobic exercise and healthy eating habits has proven to be most effective for fat loss and muscle toning. *Strength Training* for Women has been developed as a training guide as more women begin to understand the health benefits of this activity. A series of strength training routines for use in the gym as well as a body weight workout routine that can be performed at home are included.

144 pages, full-color print
200 color photos
Paperback, 6^{1}/2" x 9^{1}/4"
ISBN: 9781841262482
$ 14.95 US / $ 22.95 AUS
£ 9.95 UK/€ 14.95

Paul Collins
Speed for Sport

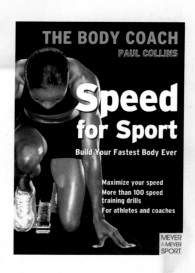

Speed is the number one factor linked to improving athletic performance in sport. Paul Collins' unique coaching guides you step-by-step through increasing speed for sport. The book offers over 100 of the latest speed training drills used by world class athletes and sporting teams for developing speed, agility, reaction and quickness.

208 pages, full-color print,
285 photos, 11 illustr., 4 charts
Paperback, 6^{1}/2" x 9^{1}/4"
ISBN: 9781841262611
$ 17.95 US / $ 32.95 AUS
£ 14.95 UK/€ 17.95

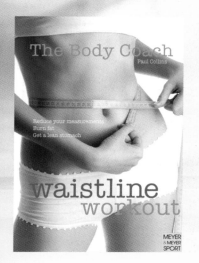

Paul Collins
Waistline Workout

The *Waistline Workout* works like magic, as The Body Coach® Paul Collins, Australia's Personal Trainer™, takes the guesswork out of dieting and exercise and guides you through his revolutionary 3-step weight loss system for achieving a slimmer and trimmer body. In a nutshell, the *Waistline Workout*, is a simple, easy-to-follow roadmap to healthy eating, proper exercise and increasing your energy levels with an 12-week workout plan.

136 pages, full color print
129 color photos, 19 charts
Paperback, 6 ^{1}/2" x 9 ^{1}/4"
ISBN: 9781841262857
$ 14.95 US / $ 22.95 AUS
£ 9.95 UK/€ 14.95

MEYER & MEYER Sport | www.m-m-sports.com
sales@m-m-sports.com

MEYER
& MEYER
SPORT

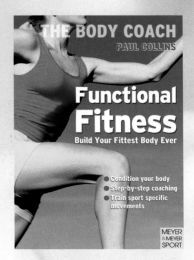

Paul Collins
Functional Fitness

Functional Fitness features practical, easy-to-follow exercises for athletes, coaches and fitness enthusiasts in helping build your fittest body ever by simulating sports-specific and daily lifestyle movement patterns.

The Body Coach®, Paul Collins, provides step-by-step coaching and workouts utilizing: body weight, fitness balls, medicine balls, plyometrics, resistance bands, stability training and speed training equipment.

144 pages, full-color print
332 photos, 9 illustr., 3 charts
Paperback, $6^1/2$" x $9^1/4$"
ISBN: 9781841262604
$ 17.95 US / $ 29.95 AUS
£ 12.95 UK/€ 16.95

Paul Collins
Stretching Basics

Stretching Basics is a user-friendly exercise guide for achieving a more supple and flexible body using your own body as resistance. It provides an introductory guide for stretching and flexibility exercises for sport, lifestyle, and injury prevention. Body Coach Paul Collins provides step-by-step instructions for more then 50 exercises meant to improve flexibility and range of motion, as well as to reduce muscular tension throughout the whole body. *Stretching Basics* is ideal for all age groups and ability levels.

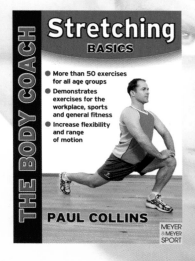

144 pages, full-color print
255 color photos
Paperback, $6^1/2$" x $9^1/4$"
ISBN: 9781841262208
$ 14.95 US / $ 22.95 AUS
£ 9.95 UK/€ 14.95

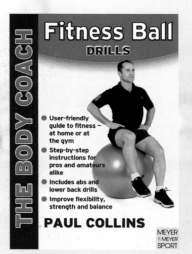

Paul Collins
Fitness Ball Drills

Fitness Ball Drills is a user-friendly exercise guide for achieving a stronger, leaner and more flexible body. The Fitness Ball is one of the most utilized pieces of gym and fitness equipment used throughout the world to tone, stretch and strengthen the whole body. Body Coach Paul Collins provides step-by-step coaching for improving posture, balance, coordination, strength and flexibility with more than 50 exercises that can easiliy be carried out at home or in the gym. *Fitness Ball Drills* is the perfect book for those who seek to improve their total body fitness.

144 pages, full-color print
182 color photos
Paperback, $6^1/2$" x $9^1/4$"
ISBN: 9781841262215
$ 14.95 US / $ 22.95 AUS
£ 9.95 UK/€ 14.95

MEYER & MEYER Sport | www.m-m-sports.com
sales@m-m-sports.com

Paul Collins
Core Strength

Core Strength features practical, easy-to-follow exercises to help you build your strongest body ever using your own body weight. The Body Coach, Paul Collins, provides step-by-step coaching with detailed descriptions of over 100 exercises. As a substitute for lifting heavy weights, *Core Strength* provides body weight exercises for strengthening, toning and reshaping every major muscle group in the body and staying in shape all year round.

200 pages, full-color print
200 color photos
Paperback, 6^1/2" x 9^1/4"
ISBN: 9781841262499
$ 17.95 US / $ 32.95 AUS
£ 14.95 UK/€ 17.95

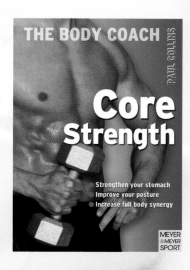

Paul Collins
Awesome Abs

The abdominal muscles serve a critical function in daily movement, sport and physical activity. A strong mid-section helps support and protect your lower back region from injury. Is packed with over 70 easy-to-follow exercises and tests aimed at achieving a leaner abdomen, a stronger lower back, better posture and a trimmer waistline. You'll not only look and feel better, but athletes will find that a well-conditioned mid-section allows them to change direction faster, generate force quicker and absorb blows better.

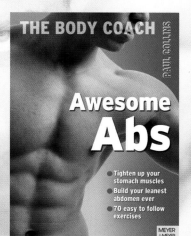

136 pages, full-color print
229 photos & 4 illustrations
Paperback, 6^1/2" x 9^1/4"
ISBN: 9781841262321
$ 14.95 US / $ 22.95 AUS
£ 9.95 UK/€ 14.95

Paul Collins
Power Training

For many years, coaches and athletes have sought to improve power, a combination of speed and strength, in order to enhance performance. *Power Training* is designed as an educational tool to assist in the development of training programs that aim to keep athletes fit, strong and powerful all year round. 80 power training drills, tests and training routines are included which have also been used by Olympic and world class athletes to improve their performance. *Power Training* is an excellent guide for conditioned athletes to increase and develop their jumping, sprinting and explosive power.

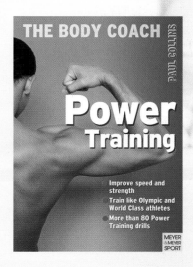

136 pages, full-color print,
247 photos
Paperback, 6^1/2" x 9^1/4"
ISBN: 9781841262338
$ 14.95 US / $ 22.95 AUS
£ 9.95 UK/€ 14.95

www.m-m-sports.com

MEYER & MEYER SPORT

photos: © Fotolia.com

Photo & Illustration Credits: